SECRETS TO A HEALTHY METABOLISM

GET SLIM, STAY SATISFIED

BY: MARIA EMMERICH

FOREWORD BY: DR. WILLIAM DAVIS

JUNE 2012

CONTENTS

GRATITUDE

Gratitude unlocks the fullness of life.
It turns what we have into enough,
and more.

It turns denial into acceptance,
chaos into order,
confusion into clarity....

It turns problems into gifts,
failures into success,
the unexpected into perfect timing,
and mistakes into important events.

Gratitude makes sense of our past,
brings peace for today
and creates a vision for tomorrow.

CREDITS

The author of this book is Maria Emmerich and her husband Craig did the editing/publishing.

Thank you to Jamie Shultz for the cover design and photography.

FOREWORD

In Maria Emmerich's newest edition of *Secrets to a Healthy Metabolism,* she continues to unleash a barrage of hard-hitting new strategies to gain control over weight, metabolism, and overall health.

When it comes to dashing conventional notions, Maria courageously takes a scorched earth policy and clears all the nutritional clutter from the scene. Unlike the hordes of dietitians and nutritionists who continue to repeat the "cut the fat, eat more healthy whole grains" fiction propagated by Big Food industry and agribusiness, Maria charts an entirely new course in eating to reset metabolism, showing the reader how to use proteins and fats to metabolic advantage. She is also adept at discussing nutritional supplements and how they can be used to complement an effective nutrition program. She provides plenty of scientific rationale for her arguments.

Maria's approach demonstrates a critical principle: Health and weight loss are not the primary goals; they are important *side-benefits* that accompany regaining control over healthy metabolism. In other words, the metabolic mess that most people begin with must first be corrected. Once achieved, healthy metabolism *allows* weight loss and health to proceed.

Maria also takes the reader down the path of getting started on wheat-free foods and baking. This area is especially challenging and Maria is the Grand Master of Wheat-free Baking! Although Secrets to a Healthy Metabolism is not a cookbook, the section on wheat-free alternative ingredients alone is invaluable.

Having gone down a similar path as Maria, having witnessed the weight gain and poor health that results from a low-fat, high-carbohydrate style of eating, Maria's approach is thoroughly refreshing and enlightening.
Dr. William Davis – Author of New York Times Best Seller "Wheat Belly"

CHAPTER 1

ABOUT ME

My journey from an overweight teen to a fit adult!

"I am standing by the shore of a swiftly flowing river and hear the cry of a drowning man. I jump into the cold waters. I fight against the strong current and force my way to the struggling man. I hold on hard and gradually pull him to shore. I lay him out on the bank and revive him with artificial respiration. Just when he begins to breathe, I hear another cry for help. I jump into the cold waters. I fight against the strong current, and swim forcefully to the struggling woman. I grab hold and gradually pull her to shore. I lift her out onto the bank beside the man and work to revive her with artificial respiration. Just when she begins to breathe, I hear another cry for help. I jump into the cold waters. Fighting again against the strong current, I force my way to the struggling man. I am getting tired, so with great effort I eventually pull him to shore. I lay him out on the bank and try to revive him with artificial respiration. Just when he begins to breathe, I hear another cry for help. Near exhaustion, it occurs to me that I'm so busy jumping in, pulling them to shore and applying artificial respiration that I have no time to see who is upstream pushing them all in...." (Adapted from a story told by Irving Zola).

I love this story because it demonstrates what we are doing for the health of our country. Instead of looking upstream at why the people are drowning, we are pulling them out after the problem has occurred. We need to look at the root of why so many people are obese and children are suffering from adult diseases, not put a "Band-Aid" on them once the problem has already happened.

You wouldn't put diesel in a gasoline engine and expect it to run…but that is what Americans are guilty of doing to their bodies on a daily basis. We consistently fuel our bodies with processed, pre-packaged foods that evolutionary science has proven makes our bodies stop running efficiently; and I also was guilty of this.

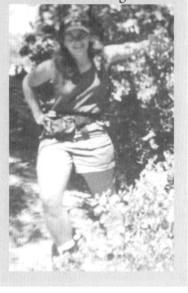

This Picture is of me on my "Fat Free" diet at age 16.

I still remember sitting in the library at age 16. I tried on my friend Lisa's jacket. All of a sudden I heard a boy sing, "fat girl in a little coat." That started my wake up call. I wanted to be like Lisa; I hated always being the fat-friend and never the girlfriend. I started skipping the afterschool trips to Tasty Treat for a gooey hot fudge sundae with the girls and replaced that with walking with my older sister. I also decided to create my own diet plan. I ate whatever I wanted for breakfast and I mean anything; my favorite was the leftover cinnamon rolls from the coffee shop I worked at. I ate a large salad for lunch with fat-free French dressing…yuck! Then diet coke for the rest of the day. Guess what? It worked, I lost weight…I felt terrible, but boys started to notice me, so I thought it was worth it.

I decided to study nutrition and exercise science in college. I met Craig (my husband) and fell in love. I started gaining the "love weight." I thought I would just kick my exercise into a higher gear; I started running and was up to 11 miles a day but I was still not losing any weight. I started running marathons and was considered a "Clydesdale" runner. What a humiliating title…it means an overweight runner that needs special cushioning shoes for the extra weight. Times Magazine wrote an article in 2009 called, "Exercise Doesn't Help with Weight Loss," which is what I was focusing on to lose fat and it wasn't working. My diet was filled with whole grain carbohydrates (for "carb-loading") and fat-free desserts.

Fat and frustrated, I finally decided to add in the nutrition part to my exercise and practice all the information I was about to preach to the world once I would graduate. I included more protein; especially for breakfast…skim milk in your Cheerio's doesn't count as a protein! I was a fat "restrictor" and exercised constantly. After decades of being told by marketing geniuses that "fat free" was the way to lose weight, eating real fat was scary for me. Once I started adding fat to my diet, I slept deeper, felt calmer and better in that first week than I ever had. Now, I understand the biochemical reasons why restricting fat is not the answer. All my life I was taught that good-tasting foods made you fat. It is almost too much to imagine that you can have total satiety while enjoying butter, avocados, grass-fed cheeses and meats, and even sugar-free cheesecake. But it has been over five years and my body feels amazing and I never feel deprived. I traded in a lifetime of over exercising and fat restriction for nutrient-dense fat-filled diet and lost weight in the process.

So why do we get mixed messages in fitness magazines and health books? Well, there are also a lot of misguided assumptions about which sources of information are objective and reliable. It is interesting that the first place magazine writers go for nutritional information is the American Dietetic Association; which has a marketing connection with the USDA and food companies that manufacture processed foods. And these companies push the foods that make the most money for them…low-fat, trans-fat junk.

I have struggled with food and weight for my whole adolescence and into adulthood. My weight loss was a hard goal to achieve, but once I found the right foods and ditched the fake foods, it became easy. I learned the secrets of the hormone insulin and the lesser known hormone leptin, that by evolving toward a very low-glycemic, high-fat (not just high-protein) diet, I had re-sensitized my biochemistry to these essential hormones, which turn off severe food cravings. Best of all, my diet makeover required a lot less self-deprivation than what I was suffering from when I wasn't losing weight. The nutrient-rich, relatively high-fat dietary approach I have developed for myself, exotic, little-known replacements for typical high-glycemic starchy foods and sugar are what finally gave me total peace with food; something I never imagined possible. The weight came off, even more than my original goal. By the end of this book, I will show you these exotic tasty weight loss foods; such as almond flour for cookies, coconut flour for cakes, after all, we also need to enjoy the sweetness of life.

When it comes to food, before coming to me for help, most of my clients have been living each day in either a temporarily "successful" state of self-deprivation or in a rebound period of gluttony. As a result, the rate of eating disorders in America is at an all-time high, as much as 65 percent. The love-hate relationship with food typically starts with innocent dieting and calorie counting, followed by out of control bingeing that causes dangerous extremes, such as skipping meals, obsessive-compulsive exercise, and purging. It is no wonder that food becomes the enemy; which is an unhappy state to be in. I help clients discover the beauty that nutrition can give us a life free from cravings and weight gain if we choose the right items.

Before my revelation of the biochemistry of food and our weight, I was so proud of my "perfect" diet of whole grains, fruits, and fat-free desserts, but I was still puzzled why I had uncontrollable cravings around food. By finding the correct supplements to change my biochemical imbalances, I started a high healthy-fat, grain-free, no starch diet; I finally found peace in my body. I didn't feel deprived or compelled to overeat.

The 'secret' is to control leptin and insulin hormones. Any diet that stops blood sugar and insulin spikes also allows the cells to regain sensitivity to the noteworthy anti-aging, weight and hunger-regulating hormone called leptin. The hardest part is to get my clients to not be afraid of fat because it is almost impossible to obtain this effect without significant amounts of fat in the diet. High protein alone doesn't work because excess protein will also turn to sugar. Low fat, high protein diets will fail to keep your blood sugar from spiking, and will not allow your leptin hormone to increase. Ron Rosedale, MD, author of The Rosedale Diet and a pioneering scientist on the hormone leptin, states, "If you don't get enough fat, you will likely eat too much protein, which then turns to sugar."

I am writing this book to everyone who has been frustrated with the way they feel, inside and out. Maybe you look great, but nutrition isn't enhancing how you feel intrinsically. Nutrition is a huge part of how we feel and operate every day. I love feeling energetic and confident and I want you to also. I was miserable when I constantly deprived myself and felt guilty when I ate. The dumbest thing I did was make "fat-free" desserts filled with junk like fat-free cool-whip, fat-free cream cheese, pudding…yuck. I want you to also find peace and enjoyment with real food; which can turn into holistic peace in your everyday life.

The way I was eating was setting me up for a whole array of issues. Here are some common problems with a diet filled with pre-packaged junk stuffed into cereal boxes and fat-free dressings:

Body Part	What Happens	What's the Problem?
Bones	Weak bones, osteoporosis	Lack of protein & omega 3 fats & consuming phytates
Energy Level	Anemia (tired all the time)	Gluten allergy, lack of vitamin E, K, iron, zinc, B_6, or B_{12},
Eyes	Dark circles under eyes	Not enough iron (red meat) or gluten allergy
Gastrointestinal tract	Irritable Bowel Syndrome	Lack of Fiber, or low good gut bacteria
Hair	Depigmentation (gray hair), slow hair growth	Not enough protein
Hair	Hair loss	Not enough biotin, iron, B6, B12, or folate (protein), food allergy!
Hair	Dry and brittle hair	Not enough iodine
Mouth	Cracked lips; swollen, dark red tongue	Not enough vitamin B2
Skin	Dry, scaly, old-looking skin	Not enough essential fatty acids, vitamin E, or protein
Skin	Varicose veins	Too much salt and sugar
Skin	Acne or "Back-acne"	Lack of zinc (protein), vitamin A and C, omega 3's.
Skin	Rosacea	Lack of vitamin B3, C, zinc, and healthy omega 6 oils.
Soft tissues	Delayed wound healing	Not enough vitamin A, vitamin C, or zinc (protein)
Hormone imbalance	Restless leg syndrome, leads to lack of sleep	Lack of iron and magnesium

So often we focus on calorie reduction for weight loss because we are told metabolism comes down to calories in, calories out. This is really only one piece of the puzzle. If you are eating 500 calories of carbohydrates at a meal you are going to be storing a lot more fat. However, if those 500 calories are a combination of protein, carbohydrates, and fat, you could actually burn fat!

Sadly, the food industry has been adding empty calories to traditional foods. In the early 1970's, food manufacturers started adding a cheap substance to foods…high fructose corn syrup. Corn is cheap and abundant, and thanks to government subsidies, Americans desire for sweets has increased tenfold. Over the past fifteen years, our food industry has increased products filled with carbohydrates; such as adding unneeded sweeteners to marinara sauce, baby formula, ketchup, yogurts, and chicken breasts. Yes, I said chicken breasts. McDonald's grilled chicken breast ingredients list is: *Chicken breast filets with rib meat, water, seasoning (salt, sugar, food starch-modified, maltodextrin, spices, dextrose, autolyzed yeast extract, hydrolyzed [corn gluten, soy, wheat gluten] proteins, garlic powder, paprika, chicken fat, chicken broth, natural flavors (plant and animal source), caramel color, polysorbate 80, xanthan gum, onion powder, extractives of paprika), modified potato starch, and sodium phosphates.* WHAT a joke! **Here's a terrifying statistic; the average piece of chicken's protein content has dropped by a third since 1971!**

We're relentlessly told that carbohydrates are the good guys of nutrition, and that, if we eat large amounts of them, the world will be a better place. The "food pyramid" tell us, there will be no heart disease and no obesity. With these words of wisdom, Americans are gobbling cereals, breads and pastas as if they were preparing for a marathon, trying desperately to reach that 75 to 85% of total calories advocated by the high-carb fanatics.

This is creating a terrible paradox: people are eating less fat and getting fatter! Overeating carbohydrate foods can prevent a higher percentage of fats from being used for energy, and lead to a decrease in endurance and an increase in fat storage. There is an alarming conclusion discovered: a high-carbohydrate, low-fat diet may be dangerous to your health.

Eating fat does not make you fat. It's your body's response to excess carbohydrates in your diet that makes you gain weight. Your body has a limited capacity to store excess carbohydrates, but it can easily convert those excess carbohydrates into excess body fat.

It's hard to lose weight by simply restricting calories. Eating less and losing excess body fat do not necessarily go hand in hand. Low-calorie, high-carbohydrate diets generate a series of biochemical signals in your body that will take you out of the balance, making it more difficult to access stored body fat for energy. As a result, you will reach a weight-loss plateau, beyond which you simply can't lose any more weight.

People on restrictive diets get tired of feeling hungry and deprived. Diets based on calorie limits and choice restriction usually fails. People are unsatisfied, go off their diets, put the weight back on as increased body fat, and then feel like a failure for not having enough will power or discipline.

A recent Harvard University study found that people who had the highest saturated fat intake also had the *least* plaque buildup on their artery walls. The *American Journal of Clinical Nutrition* described the findings as an "American Paradox." In a Stanford University study that made recent headlines, women on the "fatty" Atkins diet ended up with the healthiest cholesterol levels and the best blood pressure readings, compared to those on other diets, notably the famous high-carb low-fat diet. Since the 1970s, American men have decreased their saturated fat intake by 14% and increased their carbohydrate intake by 23% --yet rates of obesity and heart disease are increasing. The more carbs you eat, the higher your insulin levels climb, which signals your liver to produce saturated fat. If you go on a healthy-carb diet, your insulin levels drop, and so does production of saturated fat.

The success to weight loss has little to do with discipline. You need the proper information to make powerful changes. People need to focus on WHAT to eat rather than HOW MUCH. Eating a diet of low carbohydrate meals, you can eat enough to feel satisfied and still wind up losing fat-without obsessively counting calories or fat grams.

Sadly, many people don't really know what a carbohydrate is. Most people will say carbohydrates are sweets and pasta. They often think that a vegetable or fruit as a food type all its own; a food that they can eat in unlimited amounts without gaining weight. This may come as a surprise, but sweets and pasta, vegetables and fruits are all carbohydrates. Carbohydrates are merely different forms of simple sugars linked together in polymers. We all need a certain amount of carbohydrates in our diet. The body requires a continual intake of carbohydrates to feed the brain, which uses glucose as its primary energy source. In fact, the brain is a virtual glucose hog, gobbling more than two thirds of your carbohydrate stores in the bloodstream while you are at rest. To feed this glucose hog, the body constantly takes carbohydrates and converts them to glucose.

The process is a bit more in-depth than that. Any carbohydrates not immediately used by the body will be stored in the form of glycogen. The body has two storage sites for glycogen: the muscles and the liver. The glycogen stored in the muscles is inaccessible to the brain. Only the glycogen stored in the liver can be sent back to the bloodstream so as to maintain adequate blood sugar levels for proper brain function. The liver's capacity to store carbohydrates in the form of glycogen is very limited and can be easily depleted within ten to twelve hours. So the liver's glycogen reserves must be maintained on a continual basis. That's why we eat carbohydrates. The trick is to choose the right ones to sustain our blood sugar levels for the optimal time.

What happens when you eat too many carbohydrates? No matter where the carbohydrates are being stored, liver or the muscles; the total storage capacity of the body for carbohydrate is really quite limited. If you're an average person, you can store about three hundred to four hundred grams of carbohydrate in your muscles, but you can't use that carbohydrate. **In the liver, where carbohydrates are accessible for glucose conversion, you can store only about 60-90 grams. This is equivalent to about two cups of cooked pasta or three bananas.**

Once the levels in the liver are filled with glycogen, excess carbohydrates have just one fate: to be converted into fat and stored. Even though carbohydrates are fat-free, excess carbohydrates ends up as excess fat. But that's not the worst of it. Any meal or snack high in carbohydrates will generate a rapid rise in blood glucose. To adjust for this rapid rise, the pancreas secretes the hormone insulin into the bloodstream. Insulin then lowers the levels of blood glucose. **The problem is that insulin is mainly a storage hormone; it works to put aside excess carbohydrate calories in the form of fat in case of a future food shortage. The insulin that's stimulated by too many carbohydrates assertively promotes the accumulation of body fat. To recap, when we eat too much carbohydrate, we are sending a hormonal message, through insulin, to the body that states: "Store as fat".** They also tell it not to release any stored fat. When this happens, you can't use your own stored body fat for energy. So the excess carbohydrates in your diet not only make you fat, they make sure you stay fat.

After you eat carbohydrates your pancreas releases insulin and your blood sugar increases. Insulin makes sure your cells receive some blood sugar necessary for life, and increases glycogen storage. But, it also tells your body to use more carbohydrate, and less fat, as fuel. Insulin also converts almost half of your carbohydrate intake to fat for storage in-case of an energy emergency. If you want to burn fat for energy, the insulin response must be decreased. Eating refined sugars release a lot of insulin, allowing less stored fat to be burned.

High insulin levels also suppress two important hormones: growth hormone and glucagon. Growth hormone is used for muscle development and building new muscle mass. Glucagon promotes the burning of fat and sugar. Eating a high carbohydrate meal also stimulates hunger. As blood sugar increases, insulin rises with an immediate drop in blood sugar. This results in hunger, often only a couple of hours after the meal. Cravings, usually for sweets, are frequently part of this cycle, leading you to snack on more carbohydrates. Not eating makes you feel ravenous shaky, moody and ready to "crash." This cycle causes you to never get rid of that extra stored fat, and a decrease in energy.

Does this sound like you? The best suggestion for anyone wanting to utilize more fats is to moderate the insulin response by limiting the intake of refined sugars, and keeping all other carbohydrate intake to less than 30% of the diet. I have eliminated all grains from my diet and have never felt better. That means no pasta, rice, oatmeal, cereal, the government recommended "whole grains" and all. I get my carbohydrates with nutrient packed non-starchy veggies, nuts and seeds. Proteins and fats-don't produce much insulin. Eating protein and fat while eating carbohydrates can slow the increase in blood sugars down significantly.

Insulin responses are different in everybody. However, refined foods increase insulin reactions. The main reason is that refined carbohydrates lack the natural fiber which helps minimize the insulin response. Eating natural fiber with carbohydrates can reduce the blood sugar reactions described above. Low-fat diets cause quicker digestion and absorption of carbohydrates in the form of sugar. By always adding some fats to your diet, you will slow down digestion and absorption, and the insulin reaction won't be so extreme. Decreasing refined carbohydrates and increasing fats will help bring your body back into balance. By moderating carbohydrate intake you can increase your fat burning as an optimal fuel source.

We evolved for hundreds of thousands of years from the so-called "cave man's diet," which consisted of meat and vegetables. With the onset of modern civilization, our physiology suddenly was asked to digest and metabolize larger amounts of starch and refined sugars. We are unable to utilize the amount of carbohydrates we eat; therefore, certain symptoms develop.

OVERCONSUMPTION OF REFINED CARBOHYDRATES:

1. **Fatigue:** The most common feature of Insulin Resistance is that it makes people exhausted. Some are tired only in the morning or afternoon; others are wiped all day.

2. **Brain fog:** Insulin Resistance is often mental. Not being able to concentrate is the most evident symptom. Poor memory, failing or poor grades in school are often a side effect of Insulin Resistance. Are you sending your kids off to school with a bowl of cereal and skim milk??? Not a good idea.

3. **Low blood sugar.** Feeling jittery and moody is common in Insulin Resistance, with an immediate relief once food is eaten. Dizziness is also caused by low blood sugar, as is the craving for sweets.

4. **Intestinal bloating.** Most intestinal gas is produced from too many carbohydrates. People with Insulin Resistance who eat carbohydrates suffer from gas, lots of it. Antacids or other remedies for symptomatic relief are not very successful in dealing with the problem.

5. **Tired After Meals**. Being sleepy after meals containing more than 20% or 30% carbohydrates is a main side-effect. This is typically a pasta meal, or even a meat meal which includes bread or potatoes and a sweet dessert.

6. **Increased fat storage and weight**. In males, a large abdomen is the more evident and earliest sign of Insulin Resistance. In females, it is stored in the hips and thighs.

7. **Increased triglycerides**. Even normal weight individuals may have stores of fat in their arteries as a result of Insulin Resistance.

8. **Increased blood pressure**. Doctors now recognize that most people with hypertension have too much insulin and are Insulin Resistant. There is often a direct relationship between the level of insulin and the level of blood pressure: as insulin levels increase, so does blood pressure.

9. **Depression**. Carbohydrates are a natural "downer," depressing the brain; it is not uncommon to see many depressed persons also having Insulin Resistance. Carbohydrates change the brain chemistry. Carbohydrates produce a depressing or 'tired' feeling. On the flip side, protein is a brain stimulant, picking you up mentally.

10. **Alcoholism**: Insulin Resistance is also prevalent in people addicted to alcohol, caffeine, cigarettes or other drugs. Often, the alcohol is the secondary problem, with Insulin Resistance being the primary one. Alcohol becomes sugar in our bodies. This is why recovering alcoholics often overeats sweets, which causes a relapse…we never kicked the true addiction…sugar!

HOW TO BECOME BALANCED

1. **Protein**. Know how much protein your body needs. Don't consume more protein than your body requires, but more importantly, never consume less. Finding your balance can be tricky. On average, protein requirements range from 60 grams per day for a sedentary obese individual to as much as 200 grams per day for a lean heavily exercising athlete. You should have protein in EVERY meal to help balance hormone levels.

2. **Carbohydrates**. You should also choose your carbohydrates wisely. If you are insulin resistant, have high blood pressure, high cholesterol, high blood pressure or are overweight then you need to specifically restrict your carbohydrates to low starch vegetables, low sugar fruits and whole grains

filled with fiber. Starchy-refined carbohydrates cause inflammation in our body which aggravates existing health issues. If you find yourself hungry and craving sugar two to three hours after a meal, you probably ate too many carbohydrates in the previous meal. If you have a problem with hunger or carbohydrate cravings, look at what you ate for a clue to the problem. Decrease the amount of carbohydrates and increase the amount of protein.

3. **Fat.** Coconut oil and fish are great choices. Healthy fats help balance out hormone levels and decrease inflammation. Stick with natural fats; such as butter and cheese. Think about eating as natural as possible. "American" cheese is anything but natural! Fat also is essential to decrease the fat storing hormone, insulin.

4. **Water.** Try to drink half your body weight in ounces per day. The liver produces bile to break down fat, but if the kidneys are dehydrated, the liver stops its main job to help out the kidneys. Hydrated cells balance hormone levels. Caffeine tends to increase insulin levels, so go easy on the coffee.

5. **Exercise.** Exercise is very helpful for balancing insulin levels. Try to get 30 to 60 minutes of walking most days a week.

INSULIN
___

This figure shows how Insulin affects the different functions of the human body.

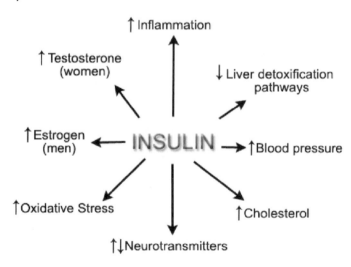

CHAPTER 2

WHAT IS METABOLISM?

THE SCIENCE OF METABOLISM

I know as a writer, you need to "capture" your audience; so please stay awake. I need to start like Mr. Gibbon (my biology teacher) and start off with the definition of metabolism. Metabolism consists of all "the chemical processes occurring within a living cell or organism that are necessary for the maintenance of life." To frustrated dieters, however, metabolism has come to refer more narrowly to the merciless calculus of calories. Metabolism is the body's natural process of converting the calorie intake from the foods you eat into energy. Many people have the misconception about metabolism and believe they are stuck with the metabolic rates they have right now and that it is an unchanging factor you were born with. You will discover that you are in the driver seat and are able to change that. It took me years to discover this power.

We have all heard this before: Take in fewer calories than we use and we'll lose weight. Take in more and we'll gain it. You don't need to read a book, "Weight loss for Dummies" to know this. It is drilled into our head during our first attempts at dieting. But there is a lot more to consider. Let's start with the three pieces that make up our metabolism. Let's imagine a pie chart...

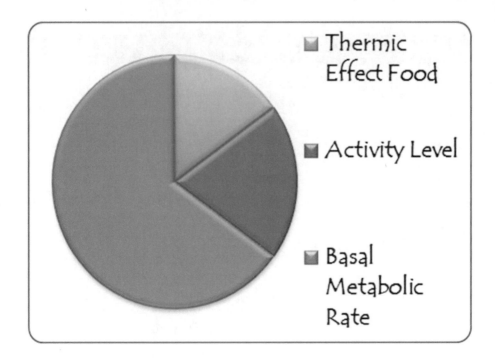

1. BASAL METABOLIC RATE (BMR)

The scientific definition of BMR is "the energy expended when an individual is lying at complete rest, in the morning, after sleep, in the post-absorptive state." BMR is around 60 to 70 percent of our daily metabolism and by far the largest piece of the pie. Our BMRs have many functions; such as, immune response, blood circulation, lung function and tissue repair. For example, **severe burn victims have had BMRs exceeding 8,000 calories a day while lying motionless** on hospital beds. Even recovering from the flu or a common cold expends a huge number of calories. This is also why smokers often gain weight after they quit; their bodies are trying to repair the damaged cells and lungs so they have a higher metabolism. This is no reason to start on the "cancer sticks," smoking also adds so many toxins into our body, the liver can't function efficiently (see Toxic Liver chapter).

Here's where we can make some changes to our metabolism. Three-quarters of variability of our BMR is determined by lean body mass. Our lean body mass includes our bones and organs, which we can't change, but it also includes our muscles, which we are in total control of their fate! As we get older, it is extremely important to maintain and build our muscles.

There is a phenomenon called sarcopenia that happens with age. Sarcopenia causes us to lose 1 percent of muscle a year starting around age 25 and most of us replace this valuable muscle with fat.

Many of us boast that we could eat anything in the past and not gain a pound, but that things have changed. Having busy jobs, families and other distractions that keep up from staying active and full of muscle have changed our abilities to burn those calories.

2. THERMIC EFFECT OF FOOD (TEF)

The thermic effect of food is a new term to many people. I refer to it as TEF. It is the caloric "handling cost" of using, digesting and storing food energy. This is also somewhat in your control. It is determined a little bit by your genes, but it also is determined by your dietary preferences. TEF can vary from 10 to 15 percent of total metabolism. So when you eat a meal that consists of a 1,000-calories your body is actually absorbing only 850 to 900. I noted that you are somewhat in charge of this. If you eat 100 calorie "snack pack," you will consume 100 calories. Your body doesn't need to work to burn this off. On the other hand, if you consume 100 calories of chicken, your body turns up the heat because of the nitrogen in protein; therefore you absorb fewer calories, your glucagon hormone kicks in and your metabolism starts to fire!

Our TEF works with the digestive system to break down food into building blocks. Carbohydrates (simple and complex) are reduced to simple sugars, fats to fatty acids, and proteins to amino acids. These building blocks enter the bloodstream and circulate throughout the body, and are essential for our bodies to work properly. Inside each cell, tiny powerhouses called mitochondria break down food molecules and tap their energy into forms, such as ATP and creatine phosphate, which give us energy and life for our bodies.

3. ACTIVITY LEVEL

Metabolism's third and most controllable "piece of the pie" is our activity level. This includes planned activity; such as running on a treadmill; as well as unconscious movements that we perform daily; such as tapping your foot in a meeting. Our activity level makes up 15 to 30 percent of our metabolism.

This piece of the pie is often way over appreciated. We often console our bodies with food after a hard workout. To put in perspective; a runner burns about 2,600 calories during a marathon and it takes 3,500 calories to burn one pound of fat...check out Times Magazine Article online: "Exercise Doesn't Help You Lose Weight." The average person is busy with family and is lucky to get in three, one-hour workouts a week. To put that in perspective that is only 2 percent of your week. I'm not trying to discourage you; I just want you to be aware that unplanned activity can add up really fast. Going to the grocery store and cooking dinner can burn as many calories as running on a boring treadmill for 40 minutes.

So instead of going to the gym after work and then stress out on the way home because you don't have anything planned for dinner so you stop at Applebee's car-side to go; go to the grocery store, power shop and make your family a healthy meal! AND there is no need to complain that healthy eating costs so much because you just saved a ton by not buying frozen junk food heated up at a restaurant. It is all about priorities, we don't blink an eye when we pay $20 for a restaurant pizza, but $12 for a free range chicken is too much...this is the wrong mentality for a healthy body.

My mom often reminds me that her grandparents always had dessert. I remind her that they worked on a farm all day. Could you imagine their faces if they saw people running on a stationary piece of metal staring at a TV for an hour? Oh yeah, they also made their pies with real fats and sugar, not Crisco and high fructose corn syrup! So get off the couch and increase your unplanned activity. Start wearing a pedometer and I'm sure you will surprise yourself at just how many extra steps you will start taking.

Do I exercise? Yes, I run, bike, walk, lift weights, practice yoga...I LOVE to move, but I did all this when I was fat too. Nutrition was the key that I was missing to successful weight loss.

CHAPTER 3

HOW TO EAT

No, I am not going to tell you that 70% of Americans don't get enough "whole grains" like the commercials on TV do. The government subsidized foods are to the United States as the oil industry is to Saudi Arabia. The US needs people to believe this lie in order to keep the money flowing.

Eat more protein

The most important piece of our thermic effect of food metabolism is the amount of quality protein in our diets; which influences weight loss. Protein helps us sustain muscle during weight loss, improve muscle strength and endurance, improve immunity, enhance antioxidant function, build HDL cholesterol, and helps insulin and leptin functions; all of which will help maximize our metabolism. I see a lot of clients come to me after trying Weight Watchers, which worked for a while, but they are stuck at a weight they are still uncomfortable at. Counting points isn't helpful for our biochemistry…they concentrate on calories. Saving up all your points for a Blizzard at Dairy Queen isn't going to enhance your physique; even if you only eat 800 calories a day…it is 800 calories of trans-fat filled sugar! I want to understand the science behind giving 5 cups of plain popcorn only 1 point; which becomes over 9 teaspoons of sugar in our blood. That increases insulin…our fat-storing hormone and kicks in other hormones that change our biochemistry causing more cravings for carbohydrates.

When dieters stop eating protein because of the high calorie count, their cells no longer contain amino acids; which gradually lowers the total lean body weight; which will cause you to lose weight. YEAH, that's good right...but think again; this affects our body composition and slows our metabolism. Because of this process we gradually need fewer calories to maintain weight. So, if the present diet is continued, weight loss will eventually stop; in fact it's even possible to slowly gain back the weight that was previously lost if a dieter faithfully sticks to a very low calorie diet! The amount of quality protein in your diet is the single most important calorie that influences your metabolism. The nitrogen in protein creates heat in our body; which increases metabolism. It also balances a lot of hormones that trigger hunger pains (see Hormone chapter). Protein helps you sustain muscle, support immune system, increase focus and concentration, and provide building blocks for neurotransmitters which provide you with a sense of well-being and energy. Do you have cravings for sugar and carbohydrates? Protein will help to decrease those as well!

For protein to be converted into amino acids or for it to repair and build cells requires a complex breakdown. This conversion uses calories; if fact, up to 30% of the calories the protein contains. Let's look at one cup of white boneless chicken breast, without the skin, contains about 230 calories 175 of those from protein. Your body will use about 30% of the calories from protein to break it down just for use. That equates to about 50 calories burned just by taking in this high-protein food. This is the thermic effect of food. Reminder: this doesn't happen with 100 calorie snack packs!

Besides burning calories as the proteins are converted, it increases your metabolism by rebuilding muscle fibers faster. Muscles require more energy, or calories, to be maintained, even when you are not using them. The more calories your body burns, the higher your metabolism.

Eating fish can increase the thermic effect of food even more. High protein often creates images of red meat and bacon. Cottage cheese, eggs, chicken, and fish are all great sources of protein. Fish packs a double punch in raising metabolic rates. Besides the high protein content, most fish contains omega-3 fat, which has been shown to help humans burn more calories. The more calories you burn, the higher your metabolism gets. **In studies conducted at the University of Western Ontario, essential fatty acids were shown to burn off about 400 extra calories per day.**

The FDA states we need 50 grams of protein per day, about 200 calories, based on a 2000 calorie diet. This guide is based on our need for nitrogen balance. Nitrogen, found only in protein, is an essential molecule required for building body structure and DNA synthesis. **The FDA's protein recommendation is only enough to help us not fade away.** Taking in only 50 grams of protein ignores the role of how protein can send our metabolism soaring. We need more protein to preserve muscle during weight loss and assist in fat burning. The FDA does not have guidelines to explain how much protein you need for exercise, stress, blood sugar support, or to help stabilize muscle as we age. So, how much do you need? The more you exercise, especially if you practice considerable weight lifting, the higher your protein intake should be, since your body tears and repairs more muscle. Weight lifters are also more at risk for catabolism, or the process of burning muscle mass for energy. A deficiency can lead to fatigue, insulin resistance, loss of muscle mass, hormone irregularities and loss of skin tone and elasticity. I suggest around 30-40 percent of calories should come from protein.

As you increase protein intake over the FDA recommendation needed for nitrogen balance, then the branch chain amino acids like leucine are also increased. Leucine is metabolized in our muscles, where other amino acids are metabolized in our liver. It benefits our muscle function and health including enhanced fat burning by muscle that unmistakably supports healthy weight loss. Research points out that during weight loss our bodies can easily lose muscle mass, and bone for that matter. Leucine has a direct signaling effect on muscle that prevents muscle loss during weight loss. This means that on a high-protein diet, the weight that is lost is mostly fat, not muscle; where on a high-carbohydrate weight-loss diet, much more muscle is lost. Leucine directly communicates to insulin, instructing it to work efficiently in muscle. This not only helps preserve your muscle mass, it helps your muscles use glucose as fuel, in turn supporting healthy insulin function. **This high-protein, leucine-rich diet consistently lowers blood levels of triglycerides, and helps leptin get into your brain easier so that you feel full on fewer calories. Once leptin gets into your brain correctly, then leptin resistance is reduced, and your metabolism gets a go signal.**

Eggs for breakfast! What about my cholesterol levels?

The most common misperception about cholesterol is that there's something unhealthy about cholesterol. Cholesterol is one of the body's repair substances: Its elevated presence in your system tells you that your body is trying to heal something; such as inflammation; which is the true source of the problem. Most Americans consume 200-300mg of cholesterol, but our body needs around 1000mg a day, so our body will produce the rest...no matter what. Our body makes extra because cholesterol is essential for hormone function, particularly the ones the body needs during stressful times. When people use statin drugs to reduce their cholesterol, instead of focusing on ridding the foods causing the inflammation (processed, fried foods) it causes muscles to deteriorate; which we know slows metabolism.

The highest sources of leucine-containing foods are animal and dairy sources. Cottage cheese, red meat, and whey protein top the list; other sources include cheese, eggs, pork, fish, chicken, peanuts, nuts, and seeds. **Eating two eggs for breakfast has been proven to boost weight loss by 65 percent, compared to the same amount of calories from carbohydrates, like a bowl of special K and skim milk.**

Eating protein for breakfast is crucial because it creates energy that outlasts carbohydrates. A boost of protein in the morning will help prevent your body from using muscle fiber for energy. Breaking down muscle for energy will slow metabolism, so it is essential that you prevent this from happening. Eating a high-protein breakfast is great for our metabolism because it wakes up our liver and gives it something to do. Your liver is the metabolic factory of your body. **A high-protein breakfast can increase your metabolic rate by 30 percent for as long as twelve hours, the calorie-burning equivalent of a 4 mile jog.** Carbohydrates are easy for your liver to use, increasing liver metabolism by only four percent, whereas protein must be taken apart and re-assembled for use in your body. This lively effect of protein has recently been shown to be the secret in supporting your natural ability to burn fat more efficiently when consuming a diet higher in protein.

Eating protein for lunch and dinner is also important to maintain muscles. A steady supply of protein throughout the day will keep that metabolism firing. If you need a snack at night, try reaching for a high-protein nibble at night, like cottage cheese or sliced turkey breast. You might find you sleep better and feel more satisfied with fewer night-time calories. High protein foods contain tryptophan, which is a natural sleep enhancer. No Tylenol PM needed. However, I don't recommend eating 3 hours before bed. If your body is metabolizing food while you sleep, you can't increase your human growth hormone; which increases our muscles and metabolism (see Human Growth Hormone chapter).

If you avoid red meat and dairy products, it harder it is to get leucine-containing foods in high amounts. Using whey protein makes it easy. Whey protein is one way to get a lot of leucine, without extra calories. I find Jay Robb brand to be the best. The flavored varieties taste great and are sweetened with Stevia, which is a no calorie sweetener. Whey protein is especially helpful in improving your brain's feeling of food satisfaction. There are many bioactive peptides in whey that regulate appetite, a benefit only attainable from consuming whey protein in higher amounts (see Whey in supplement chapter).

A higher-protein diet also has a natural diuretic effect. People with extra weight are often sluggish and holding extra water; which can cause blood pressure go up and causes our heart to push harder to move the stagnation. The extra water in connective tissues directly gets in the way of fat burning. When you eat a higher protein diet, an important blood protein called albumin increases; which, draws water back out of your connective tissues and helps you get rid of fluid retention. If you have too much inflammation, your kidneys may leak albumin into your urine, provoking fluid retention, weight problems, and considerable cardiovascular risk.

When we eat too many carbohydrates and not enough protein, the opposite happens; we retain more fluids. It also stimulates too much leptin; provoking leptin resistance and an intense desire for more carbohydrates. Too many carbohydrates cause your willpower to be in a constant battle with out-of-balance leptin. It is pretty obvious from the amount of yo-yo dieting in our culture that misguided leptin usually wins. The best way to win the battle is to not have it in the first place, meaning don't eat too many carbohydrates and more importantly, not by themselves.

PROTEIN STUDIES:

A study of 95 men and 32 women used whey protein meal replacement with 15 grams for two meals a day for six months, and then reduced to one meal replacement for six more months. While this amount of whey protein is considerably below what I and most nutritionists would recommend to assist weight loss, the results were still good. During the first six months participants lost around 20 pounds. In the next six months, on only 15 grams of whey per day, they kept their weight off and lost another 2 pounds. The participants' cardiovascular health and leptin levels were improved, including decreases in LDL cholesterol, insulin, glucose, triglycerides, and blood pressure, while HDL cholesterol increased.

Another important study was based on women with polycystic ovary syndrome (PCOS); which is a female insulin-resistance and leptin-driven endocrine predicament that can result in obesity, facial hair growth, and acne. Scientists compared a low calorie diet fortified with 60 grams of whey protein and a low calories diet with 60 grams of carbohydrates. After two-months the whey protein group lost around 20 pounds of fat, and dropped total cholesterol by 33 points, compared to the carbohydrate group which had no health increases.

Many people are under the false impression that high-protein diets are acid-forming, and therefore bad for bones. Whey protein is actually great for our bones. A study using 40 grams of whey protein per day for six months increased bone mineral density in young women by 1.57% and in postmenopausal women by 1.21%. As long as you include a well-balanced diet with plenty of fresh fruits and vegetables, and a higher protein diet, it is not bad for bones. The research tells us that low protein leads to bone loss. Fruits and vegetables create the alkaline mineral buffers so protein can support bone growth. Bone loss is common during weight loss; therefore, whey protein is a praiseworthy food to have in your pantry.

When you are sedentary, lose muscle and have compromised your health, you may have a harder time metabolizing higher amounts of protein; sedentary people in general have indigestion with most food groups. If you suffer from indigestion, gradually increase your intake while you also slowly add in physical activity. As you build strength, your pH will be better, and you will be able to reap the benefits of consuming a higher protein diet, while decreasing starchy carbohydrates. Supplemental enzymes can also assist in protein breakdown (see Supplement chapter). If you haven't eaten protein in years, your body will stop producing these enzymes and a supplement will be necessary to help rebuild proper digestion.

Fat Burning Tip:
EAT CAPSAICIN:
The high levels of capsaicin, the natural compound in the chili that makes your tongue burn, can help you to burn more calories! Studies show people who eat chilies containing capsaicin burn calories up to 15 minute longer because of all that heat that's produced in the body. Don't like spicy foods? Supplements with concentrated amounts of capsaicin are also available.

Fiber and weight loss

About 90% of my clients are looking for a quick and easy weight loss solution. Another example of foods that can speed this process is any that are high in fiber, such as veggies, flaxseeds, and nuts. When I look at a label I look at the ingredients list, but next I look at the carbohydrates and how many of those are fiber. If the fiber number is really close to the carbohydrate number, the food item is a "go."

Fiber has the ability to communicate a feeling of fullness, which can aid in weight loss. But is fiber all it's cracked up to be? Most of us have heard that fiber leads to better health, which leads to us greater pleasure in our lives. But do we know the how's, why's, and where's of fiber? This can be a confusing area of nutrition. The important part to understand is that our digestive tract is one of the most essential links to excellent health, and without fiber, also known as "roughage," your intestines have no way to clean themselves and stay healthy. Think of fiber as a "cleaning lady" for your body; no need to follow those goofy diets to clean the toxins out, just eat real food! Research reported by Harvard University correlates a high fiber diets with reduced prevalence of colon cancer, constipation, heart disease, type II diabetes, and diverticular disease.

I first learned about the benefits of fiber from Betsy Barret, an undergraduate nutrition professor. My favorite part was when she brought up a slide that stated "FIBER HAS NO CALORIES!" She went on to inform us that humans lack an enzyme that allows us to absorb the calories in fiber and use it as energy. Wow, that was a great day! I went out and bought all the fruits and veggies I knew that were filled with fiber. I wanted to always feel full, so it would help me with my cravings for peanut butter cups! I think I cleared the shelves of all the prunes from the local grocery store. That was a bad idea for a variety of reasons, not only did I have to run out of Biology class, prunes are also filled with sugar. I soon learned, that there are two kinds of fiber, and that, in order for them to be helpful for weight loss, they both need to be part of a balanced meal plan with fat included…at that time I was cutting all the fat I could too…oops. No wonder I wasn't successful.

Fiber vs. Sugar: Blood Sugar and Metabolism

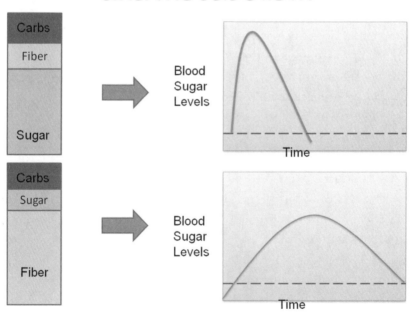

I'm sure you've heard of soluble and insoluble fiber, but how do you know which is which? Betsy, the professor, told us to imagine which parts of a whole grain, veggie or fruit would dissolve in a glass of water.

Take a pear for example; the peel is an example of insoluble fiber because it won't dissolve in water. Insoluble fiber helps prevent and relieve constipation. This type of fiber moves through the body quickly. Insoluble fiber comes from a WHOLE flaxseed, and vegetables (and grains…which you want to keep away from for many reasons). Consider insoluble fiber as a toothbrush which gently scrubs bacteria from the walls of your intestines and pushes out waste products and toxins.

Soluble fiber is when you grind the flaxseeds or the juicy pulp of the pear that does dissolve in water. Soluble fiber has been proven to decrease the risk of stroke, control blood sugar levels, and help prevent certain cancers and gastrointestinal issues. Soluble fiber also assists to lower LDL cholesterol levels and heart disease risk. Soluble fiber is found in fruits, veggies, nuts, seeds, oats, and legumes. Think of it as the sponge that soaks up excess LDL cholesterol, toxins, and bad bacteria keeping them out of your bloodstream. **Take NOTE: I do not recommend fruit, oats or legumes.**

Fiber aids in weight loss in other ways too. It helps speed our metabolism. Fiber can't be digested by the body but your body doesn't realize that. Our bodies work hard to try and use that fiber; which correlates to an increase in metabolism; as a result it burns more calories in the process.

The American Cancer Society recommends that we aim for about 25-35 grams of fiber a day, which is more than double what the average American gets. That's the equivalent of 3 heads of lettuce…yikes! If you are like most people and your daily fiber intake is less than 10 grams, be sure to increase your fiber intake slowly. Many people claim they can't eat broccoli or cauliflower because it gives them gas…well, that is because the main part of the carbohydrates in coniferous veggies is fiber (compared to a potato's carbohydrates come from a starch). They get gas because they are increasing their fiber intake too much too fast. To minimize discomfort and gas slowly increase fiber by 3-5 grams/week. Don't try to double your fiber intake while you're on a first date.

Also making sure to drink lots of water, about 8 glasses a day or until your urine is clear, to help assist the fiber through your body rather than have it just sit there. If you increase your fiber intake without increasing fluids, constipation is bound to happen. Also, if you are experiencing diarrhea, decrease your fiber intake for a few days. Some foods are high in fiber, but still too high in carbohydrates. I recommend these delicious high-fiber foods:

- Coniferous vegetables: cauliflower, broccoli, Brussels sprouts, cabbage
- Vegetable substitutes: eggplant for bread, zucchini for noodles, cauliflower for rice….are all ways to sneak fiber in.
- Flaxseeds: all the carbs come from fiber.
- Almond and Coconut Flour: great for baking
- Psyllium Husks for baked goods (see 'Alternative Flour' chapter)
- Avocado: 12 grams of fiber and tons of omega 3 fats.
- Dr. In The Kitchen's Flackers (flaxseeds, www.drinthekitchen.com)
- JUST LIKE SUGAR (see 'Sweetener' Chapter) 96g fiber/cup!!!
- **If you don't have depression, a thyroid condition or other autoimmune disease: (these contain wheat and I DON'T EAT THEM, but if you must…)**
    o Trader Joe's Sprouted Wheat Bread (4 grams of fiber per slice)
    o Damascus Flaxseed Roll-Ups (only 110 calories and 9 grams of fiber with 12 grams of protein)
    o Joseph's Lavish Bread (50 calories, 7 carbs, 4 fiber)
    o Joseph's Pita Bread (40 calories, 8 carbs, 4 fiber)

You may notice that fruit is not on the list even though it is often high in fiber. The sugar in fruit comes from fructose. Fructose makes our liver work to 80% of capacity, whereas glucose makes out liver work to 20% capacity. Raspberries, blueberries, blackberries provide 8 grams per cup and are lower in sugar, but consider these a rare treat.

Another way to tell is your food is full of fiber or not is to imagine putting a carbohydrate-rich food into your mouth, and sucking on it. Imagine a piece of white bread (don't really put white bread in your mouth ever). Does it dissolve entirely? Of course it does, because it is pure starch! Manufactures striped all the healthy benefits out of the grains. Now try a piece of avocado. What remains in your mouth when all of the starch and simple sugars dissolve? That is the fiber. Feel free to swallow, because these remnants may be the most important nutrient. Imagine if you were to do this test on broccoli, you would not get very far; this is because broccoli is high in fiber, 8 grams for 1 cup raw.

I'm also not a big fan of grains. I try to replace all the grains in our house with vegetables. For example we use "cauliflower rice" instead of brown rice. But for informational purposes; products labeled "whole grains" are made with the entire grain kernel; whether the grain remains intact as in oatmeal or it is ground to make bread, pasta or cereal. Don't be misled by wording like "100% wheat" or "multi-grain." Don't be fooled by color, either. Most 100% wheat bread is nearly identical to white bread except that brown coloring has been added to make it look more natural.

Grains like white rice, white bread and breakfast cereals have had most of their fiber and nutrients stripped away. They turn into blood sugar (glucose) so fast that, like granulated sugar; they cause a spike in our insulin level. This tells our body that plenty of energy is eagerly available and that it should stop burning fat and start storing it. The more unpleasant effect is that the insulin spike is followed by a drop in insulin level that leaves us feeling tired and hungry and wanting to eat more. The unfortunate result of this situation is that it makes us want to eat something else with high sugar content. When we do, we start the cycle all over again. This is why people who eat fat-free foods usually end up eating more calories. Eating foods with plenty of fiber will help keep our blood sugar at a more consistent level.

Why no grains? And how am I going to get fiber??? The most common whole grains are not very high in fiber to begin with.

Brown Rice = 4% (Shockingly low!)
Corn = 7%
Oats = 11%
Whole Wheat = 12%
Barley = 17%

Compare that to the vegetables I use in place of them...

Red Pepper = 25% (Sloppy Joe's Stuffed Peppers)
Kale = 33% (Kale Chips)
Mushrooms = 33% (Cowboy Chicken Casserole)
Cauliflower = 40% (Cauliflower "Rice")
Broccoli = 40% ("Loaded" Broccoli)

Eggplant = 40% (Eggplant French Fries/Breadsticks)
Spinach = 50% (Pizza Quiche)

So let's compare...

1 slice whole wheat bread = 2g of fiber, 20g carbs (starch), 100 calories

1/4 cup brown rice = 2g of fiber, 35g carbs and 170 calories

1 cup cauliflower "rice" = 2g fiber, but only 4g of carbs and 30 calories

You can get just as much fiber by substituting healthier nutrient-dense veggies for "whole grains" without the excess sugar and calories!

Fiber is found primarily in carbohydrate-rich foods, which is the main reason why we need to include a balanced amount of healthy carbohydrates daily. Plan to use your carbohydrates wisely, stay away from carbohydrates that are going to increase your insulin levels, psyllium husks are a perfect all-fiber carbohydrate. Let's pretend we had a carbohydrate budget and we needed to spend at least 30 grams of fiber from a shopping spree. Choosing carbohydrates that have most of the carbohydrates from fiber (rather than from starch – which isn't usually listed on the nutritional label) gives you more for your money. Keep in mind, if you divide your goal for the day of 30 grams between 3 meals and 1-2 snacks; you need about 6-8 grams per meal and 3-4 at snacks. Don't waste your carbohydrate shopping spree with pre-packaged instant food, make sure when choosing carbohydrates you are getting the best bang for your buck…Fiber One cereal bars are basically fiber-infused candy bars! Carbohydrates with little to no fiber are the easiest food items for our body to metabolize; therefore not increasing that thermic effect of food we talked about in Chapter One.

Fiber also helps to keep our bowel movements regular. One of the first questions I ask my clients is if they "poo" every day. Yes, it is personal, but yes it is important. I had one client that only had one bowel movement a week. Ouch! We definitely added fiber and water and probiotics to her diet.

Fiber wards off disease by grabbing toxins in our intestines, binding to them, and moving them through our colon quicker than they otherwise would. Populations that eat greater amounts of fiber-rich foods are universally healthier. People who eat a diet high in fiber are less likely to grab sugary snacks for a pick-me-up. Perhaps fiber's greatest value, however, is in helping to keep us slim by increasing our metabolism.

So, why should we include more fiber? Fiber decreases risk of certain cancers, lowers LDL cholesterol, gets rid of toxins, makes us feel full sooner and stays in our stomach longer, slowing down our rate of digestion and keeping us feeling full longer. Due to its higher fiber content, one serving of whole grain bread is more filling than two servings of white bread. Fiber also moves food through our digestive system faster so less of it is absorbed. Adding more fiber to your diet will likely help you lose weight and improve your health, but remember do it gradually; rapid increases in consumption of fiber may result in gas or diarrhea. Also, be sure to drink plenty of fluids when adding fiber to your diet. While fiber is helpful to your digestive system, without adequate fluids it can cause constipation instead of helping to eliminate it. Although fiber is not a magic bullet, a high-fiber AND low carb diet, as part of a healthy-balanced lifestyle, it can really tip the scales!

Fat Burning Tip: Drink Ice Water
Water for your body is like oil for your car. You need water for all metabolic process especially if you start consuming extra fiber. Water assists in digestion, waste excretion, circulation and even breathing. Dehydration can lead to sugar cravings, fatigue, and irritability marked by edginess. Dehydration also significantly slows down fat-burning and prevents the muscles from taking advantage of the carbs you're eating.
The more ice-cold water you drink, the more calories you burn. Drinking eight ounces of cold water can burn off an additional 9.25 calories as compared to room-temperature water; this may not seem like a lot, but it can add up to one pound a month…just by drinking ice water.

Thanks to the fat-free propaganda of the 1980's, Americans misguidedly linked all dietary fats with elevated cholesterol levels, cardiovascular problems and obesity. We reacted by radically changing our dietary habits and removed fats as much as possible. With everyone cutting the fat, you'd think we'd be skinny-mini's by now, but on the contrary, the opposite is happening! By limiting our fat intake; which is **the most effective blood sugar stabilizer**; we have increased our desire for sugar, fat-free yogurt, cookies, ice cream, bagels, bread, crackers, rice cakes, basically unnatural processed foods that are filled with high fructose corn syrup.

Even the most health conscious "foodies" went overboard with fat-free carbohydrates and became overweight in the process. It is due to the idea that refined carbohydrates; like bagels and white rice, as well as 'hyped-up' complex carbohydrates; such as whole grain bread, potatoes and corn are "free" diet foods. These foods produce a quick spike in blood sugar levels, which raises insulin; which is our fat storing hormone. Corn has a higher glycemic index than most candy bars! Too much insulin blocks the body's ability to burn stored fat for energy as well as creates a rapid fall in blood sugar levels, resulting in more hunger and then we grab more unfulfilling calories. Here's something to think about...cows are fat right? But they only consume corn and no fat... hmmm...interesting. No wonder cows are now fed corn; so they can fatten up in 6 months versus 2 years for grass-fed cows. **Here's another interesting fact: SUMO WRESTLERS EAT FAT-FREE DIETS...their staple meals are rice and sugar followed by a 2 hour nap!**

Obesity Trends* Among U.S. Adults
BRFSS, 1985
(*BMI ≥30, or ~ 30 lbs. overweight for 5' 4" person)

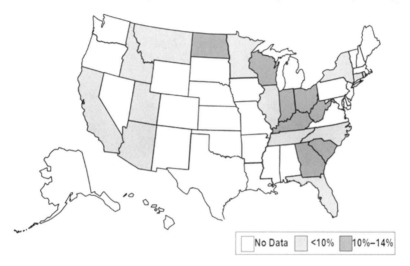

No Data | <10% | 10%–14%

BRFSS, 2009
(*BMI ≥30, or ~ 30 lbs. overweight for 5' 4" person)

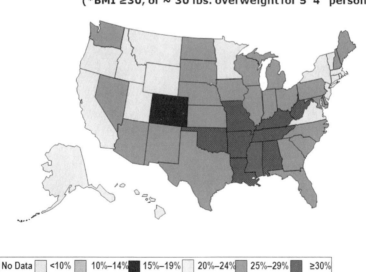

No Data | <10% | 10%–14% | 15%–19% | 20%–24% | 25%–29% | ≥30%

This roller coaster ride of blood sugar peaks and valleys has led to our national problem of weight gain. Our elimination of fat has caused our rate of obesity to skyrocket. More Americans are overweight today than ever before. Over 50% of us fall in the overweight category. And as odd as it may sound, many of these overweight individuals are suffering from a fat deficiency; specifically, an omega 3 essential fatty acid (EFA) deficiency. Essential fatty acids are 'essential' for the body's biochemical processes. **Without them, your body senses a famine and begins to convert more carbohydrates into fat, turning you into a fat-producing machine. Yikes!**

A deficiency in essential fatty acids can also cause many other problems; such as depression, ADHD, arthritis, diabetes, skin disorders, PMS and menopausal symptoms, low-energy levels, fatigue, allergies, breast cancer and yeast imbalances. Just look at the trends since Americans started cutting back the fat:

- Heart disease is now the number one killer in the US
- Diabetes have tripled in the last 30 years
- New health problems showing up (chronic fatigue, Candida, food allergies, auto-immune disorders)

A huge misperception, invented by the food industry, is that saturated fats are all bad and that trans-fatty acids are fine. The human body does not benefit from the total absence of saturated fat; that is something that medical clinicians need to learn. The heart, the kidney and muscles use saturated fats as their normal energy source. The lungs need it, as does the immune system.

In Europe and Canada people recognize that if you don't get some saturated fat in your diet it causes health problems, especially because your body can't make saturates out of trans-fat. These countries steer clear of manufactured trans-fats as much as possible. If you're consuming artificial fats and no saturated fats, you'll end up with detrimental fatty acids in the membranes. The fact is, when you start to replace the natural fats people were eating since the beginning of time with the "fats" that the food industry started creating after World War II, your body isn't going to run efficiently.

- Cancer cases have increased
- Attention Deficit Hyperactivity Disorder (ADHD) in children and adults is on the rise.

Essential fatty acids not only help your body on the inside, it also makes you "glow" on the outside. Healthy fats add luster to fragile hair, strengthen weak nails and heals skin conditions like eczema. My favorite part of fat; besides tasting SO GOOD, is that eating the right kind of fats is definitely where it's at for healthy weight loss. I know it is hard to change your mindset and enjoy fats, but believe me; when I started eating a well-balanced diet and kicked out those unfulfilling "fat-free foods" the weight started dropping. Sadly, many people have been so brainwashed by the fat-free propaganda of the past 20 years that they still suffer from fat phobia. I see client after client that struggles with adding fat to their diet. Even though it isn't working for them, the notion that all fats are bad is certainly a hard belief for them to shake.

Not all fats are created equal. There are some fats you should definitely stay away from. Hydrogenated, oxidized, fried or heat-processed fats–typically found in margarine, vegetable shortening or fried foods are sources of the unnatural and unhealthy trans-fats. These fats are linked to heart disease, cancer and aging. We all must be a detective when purchasing items at the grocery store; just because it says, "trans-fat free," isn't necessarily true. It means that it has less than one gram per serving. A serving of Coffee-mate or Cool-Whip is tiny; no one uses that small amount. Add your servings up and you might ingest 4 grams of trans-fats when you want to get 0! Always check the label for anything saying "partially hydrogenated." Even peanut butter, which I love, can have tran-fat; always choose versions that have the least ingredients: peanuts and salt! **Even one gram of trans-fat is terrible for our metabolism and it take 9 months to detox from our body!**

On the other hand, macadamia nut oil, coconut oil, flaxseed oil, fish oils, nuts, seeds, organic butter, and avocados, are protective fats that keep our blood sugar levels stable so you actually feel fuller longer. Eating these quality fats can curb food cravings and prevent overeating. Another bonus is that some of the healthy fats trigger fat burning rather than fat storage, which boosts your body's natural fat-burning ability.

The hormonal response in our body when we eat carbs/protein/fat is totally different. I am reading an interesting book of studies and this one really stood out!

1000 calories at 90% fat = 0.9 lbs lost/day
1000 calories of 90% protein = 0.6 lbs/day
1000 calories of 90% carbs = weight GAIN of .24 lbs/day

Protein creates a 'thermic effect of food,' which means that when we consume protein some calories are 'lost' as heat. Healthy fats, such as coconut oil increases thermogenesis, which increases metabolism and produces energy. The medium chain fats in coconut oil goes directly to the liver and are immediately converted to energy, we call these KETONES. It also increases metabolism because it is easily absorbed and produces organelles in our cells. So my suggestion is to cut the carbs and sugar wherever possible and up the healthy fats! The healthiest more energizing fats come from animal sources. Quality animal sources like free-range egg yolks and grass fed beef!

When you hear the words "butter" or "coconut oil" you have been trained to think "heart disease!" Well, I am here to tell you we have been replacing these natural good-mood fats with rancid vegetable oils (corn/canola/soybean) overloaded with omega 6 fats. Butter and coconut oil, actually protect the omega-3s in our brain. Outside of mother's milk, coconut oil is nature's richest source of medium chain triglycerides (MCT); they are extraordinary fats because they are not processed by your body in the same manner as long chain triglycerides.

Coconut oil increases thermogenesis, which increases metabolism and produces energy. The medium chain fats in coconut oil goes directly to the liver and are immediately converted to energy, we call these KETONES. It also increases metabolism because it is easily absorbed and produces organelles in our cells. We have studied cows and other animals with different fats:

Vegetable oils = put on weight and produce fatty meat
Coconut oil = became very lean

Normal fat metabolism depends on bile salts that have been released from your gallbladder before broken down in your digestive system. Coconut oil bypass bile metabolism and go directly to your liver where they are converted into ketones. The liver immediately releases KETONES into the bloodstream transported to the brain to be used as fuel. BENEFITS OF KETONES:

1. A stable source of energy for the brain during periods of low blood sugar without the harmful neurological side effects associated with high blood sugar.

2. Are a preferred source of brain food in people affected by diabetes or any neurodegenerative condition such as Alzheimer's, ALS, Parkinson's, & Multiple Sclerosis. In these conditions, the brain no longer uses glucose for fuel so we need to use an alternative source...ketones!

3. Help heart patients recover from a heart attack and they can dramatically shrink cancerous tumors.

4. Are proven to help decrease seizures in patients with epilepsy.

THE BALANCING ACT

Studies are showing that Americans eat too much "bad" omega-6 in the form of pre-packaged and fast food items. This creates a problem of inflammation in our body. Inflammation causes muscle loss, heart disease, high cholesterol, and acne...the list is huge. Finding a balance of omega 3s and 6s to create GLA will promote the health benefits we desire. Several issues often stop the conversion process of creating GLA; such as aging, diabetes, daily stress, smoking, viral infections, and other factors like pollution. Diets rich in sugar, trans-fats, and alcohol can also stop the necessary process of creating GLA. Because of our dietary habits, studies find that most of us are deficient in GLA. Being aware and reducing these factors whenever possible helps your body attain the benefits of the omega oils. The first thing I suggest, for a variety of reasons, is to reduce or even cut out sugar, trans-fats and alcohol. You might also consider supplementing with rich sources of GLA as well as EPA and DHA. Most Americans are somewhat familiar with fish oil containing EPA and DHA, but the omega 6, GLA, is just as important. GLA is rapidly being discovered as an immune booster, skin softener, as well as a PMS and menopause soother. Some good omega-6s have also demonstrated an ability to be awesome metabolic burners; as much as 400 calories a day (see supplement chapter; ALA and CLA).

Some really interesting studies involve obese animals. They found that both omega-3 and 'good' omega-6 oils have the ability to stop obesity. A diet loaded in fats was fed to two groups of lab mice that were obese and had diabetes. **Both groups were given the same amount of calories and fat, the slimmer mice were those given omega-3 fish oils. The fatter mice consumed unhealthy omega-6 in the form of soybean oil. The difference in their weight equated to that of a 150-pound man versus a 225-pound man! That is unbelievable!** If you want to drop those extra pounds and enjoy wide array of health benefits, put an end to your fat phobia and add healthy fats back into your diet. My clients have all been amazed at the flavorful changes. Not only did they lose weight, but their skin looked great, their hair was shiny and they had more energy.

Here's a list some dietary sources for each of these healthy fats. The key is to make sure the oils aren't processed or refined because, when that happens, the nutritional benefits of them are considerably compromised.

OMEGA-3 FAT ZAPPERS

- Macadamia Nut Oil and Nuts
- Krill Oil and Cod Liver Oil
- Walnuts (raw nuts, bottled oil or capsules)
- Pumpkin seeds
- Purslane (dark, leafy greens)
- Fatty fish (salmon, sardines, mackerel)
- Blend flaxseed oil in a protein smoothie or cottage cheese. The amino acids along with the flaxseed's fatty acids help combat breast cancer.
- Perk up your salads by using walnut oil in your dressing

    Flaxseed, flaxseed oil, and fish oils should be kept refrigerated. Whole flaxseeds must be used within 24 hours of grinding; otherwise they lose their health benefits. Also, be sure to buy omega-3 fatty acid supplements made by companies who certify that their products are free of heavy metals such as mercury, lead, and cadmium. Sam's Club's fish oils are a poor product. To check the quality of your fish oil, place your capsules in the freezer, if they freeze they have fillers and aren't quality supplements.

OMEGA-6S

- Macadamia Nut Oil and Nuts
- Pine nuts (raw nuts)
- Pistachios (raw nuts) BUT too high in starch for me!
- Sunflower seeds (raw seeds)
- Conjugated Linoleic Acid: CLA (see supplement chapter)
- 1-2 grams of borage oil daily (liquid or capsules)
- 3-6 grams of evening primrose oil (liquid or capsules)

Check labels and avoid foods with "partially hydrogenated" oils in the ingredients. When purchasing nuts, buy them raw and roast them yourself. Roasted nuts in the store have ruined the healthy properties. You'll find "bad" omega 6 trans-fats in a variety of packaged foods, like bread and crackers. Also steer clear of refined, nutrient-deficient forms of omega-6s found in corn, safflower, sunflower, soybean, and cottonseed oils...check your salad dressing bottles!

OMEGA-9S

- Sesame oil (bottled oil)
- Avocado
- Peanuts (raw or peanut oil)
- Almonds (raw) or Almond Oil
- Pecans (raw)
- Cashews (raw), but they are higher in starch/sugar!
- Hazelnuts (raw or oil form)
- Macadamia (raw or in oil form)

BENEFITS OF OMEGA 3'S:

1. **Heart disease:** Clinical evidence suggests that EPA and DHA found in fish oil help reduce risk factors for heart disease including high cholesterol and high blood pressure. Strong evidence shows that EPA and DHA can help prevent and treat atherosclerosis by reduce the build-up of plaque and blood clots, which clog arteries. Clinical studies of heart attack survivors have found that daily omega-3 fatty acid supplements significantly reduce the risk of death, additional heart attacks, and stroke.

2. **High cholesterol:** People who follow a Mediterranean-style diet tend to have higher HDL cholesterol levels. Similar to a Mediterranean diet, Inuit Eskimos consume high amounts of omega-3 fatty acids from fatty fish and have higher HDL cholesterol and lower triglyceride levels.

3. **High blood pressure:** Numerous scientific studies find that diets rich in omega-3 fatty acids lowers blood pressure considerably in individuals with hypertension. Supplementation with 3 or more grams of fish oil daily can reduce blood pressure in individuals with untreated hypertension.

4. **Diabetes:** Patients with diabetes are likely to have high triglyceride and low HDL levels. Omega-3 fatty acids from fish oil can help lower triglycerides, which is a sign of diabetes. Eating foods or taking supplements that contain DHA and EPA can help tremendously. There have been reports of small increases in fasting blood sugar levels in patients with type 2 diabetes while taking fish oil supplements.

5. **Weight loss:** As noted earlier, there is a connection between our weight and issues such as poor blood sugar control, diabetes, and high cholesterol. Clinical studies suggest that overweight people who follow a weight loss program that includes exercise tend to achieve better control over their blood sugar and cholesterol levels when omega-3 fatty acids are included in their diet.

6. **Attention deficit/hyperactivity disorder (ADHD):** I have many clients that see remarkable results with adding Omega 3's to their children's diets. Children with attention ADHD usually have low levels of certain essential fatty acids in their bodies. In a clinical study of nearly 100 boys, those with lower levels of omega-3 fatty acids had more learning and behavioral problems, such as temper tantrums and sleep disturbances, than boys with normal omega-3 fatty acid levels. Studies found large improvements in reading, spelling, and behavior in the children over 3 months of therapy. Other studies found that omega-3 fatty acid supplementation helped to decrease physical aggression in school children with ADHD.

7. **Arthritis:** Studies examining the use of omega-3 fatty acid supplements for inflammatory joint conditions have focused almost entirely on rheumatoid arthritis. Numerous studies find that omega-3 fatty acid supplements reduce tenderness in joints, decrease morning stiffness,

and decrease the amount of pharmaceutical medication needed for people with rheumatoid arthritis.

8. **Osteoporosis:** Omega-3 fatty acids help increase levels of calcium in our body, deposit calcium in the bones, and improve bone strength. Studies also suggest that people who are deficient in certain essential fatty acids, mostly the omega-6 GLA, are more likely to suffer from bone loss than those with normal levels. In a study of women over 65 with osteoporosis, those given EPA and GLA supplements experienced less bone loss over 3 years than those who were given a placebo. Many of these women also had an increase in bone density.

9. **Depression:** No wonder we get the blues on a fat-free diet. Omega-3 fatty acids are vital pieces of nerve cell membranes. They help nerve cells communicate with each other, which is a fundamental step in achieving good mental health. Levels of omega-3 fatty acids were found to be very low and omega-6 fatty acids were extremely high in a clinical study of patients hospitalized for depression. In a controlled study of patients with depression, those who ate a healthy diet consisting of fatty fish 2 - 3 times per week for 5 years experienced a significant reduction in depression and aggression.

10. **Bipolar disorder and Schizophrenia:** In a clinical study of 30 people with bipolar disorder, those who were treated with EPA and DHA, along with their prescription medications, for 4 months experienced fewer mood swings and recurrence of depression and mania than those who were given a placebo. Clinical evidence also suggests that people with schizophrenia experience an improvement in symptoms when given omega-3 fatty acids.

11. **Menstrual pain:** In a clinical study of nearly 200 Danish women, those with the highest dietary intake of omega-3 fatty acids had the mildest symptoms; decreasing cramps, hot flashes and sweating during menstruation.

12. **Skin disorders:** Many doctors believe that flaxseed is helpful for treating acne. GLA is extremely beneficial for people experiencing dry skin, eczema and dandruff.

13. **Asthma:** Omega-3 supplements (in the form of perilla seed oil, which is rich in ALA) may decrease inflammation and help lung function in adults with asthma. Too much omega-6 fatty acids have the opposite

effect; they increase inflammation and aggravate respiratory function. Taking a fish oil supplements rich in EPA and DHA is extremely helpful.

14. **Inflammatory bowel disease:** Omega-3 fatty acids may reduce symptoms of Crohn's disease and colitis. ALA is the best version of omegas for IBD.

My new favorite oil is macadamia nut oil. This oil has a high smoke point of around 425 degrees Fahrenheit. This is much higher than that of olive oil. I never fry in olive oil, I only use macadamia or coconut oil; they don't break down to products that are unhealthy for the heart. Due to its chemical structure and high amount of unsaturated fats, heating olive oil = oxidative damage. Are you leaving your bottle of olive oil right on the counter? Opening and closing it multiple times a week? Any time the olive oil is exposed to air and/or light, it oxidizes. The chlorophyll in olive oil accelerates the oxidation. Oxidation causes free radicals, which increase cancer and atherosclerosis; which are "free radical" diseases. Cancer is associated with chromosomal defects and oncogene activation. The consumption of oxidized fats and oils increase death rates from leukemia and malignant neoplasia of the breast, ovaries and rectum. Atherosclerosis increases as free radical reactions from diet-derived fats in the arterial wall increases. These compounds induce endothelial cell damage and produce changes in the arterial walls. The WORST Oils for this is: Canola, Corn, Cottonseed, Soy, Sunflower Oil, which are found in microwave dinners, salad dressings, chips, cookies, crackers, roasted nuts and most pre-packaged foods.

On the other hand, macadamia nut oil has a long shelf life. It can be stored for up to 1 to 2 years without refrigeration. Macadamia nut oil has linoleic acid, Omega-3 essential fatty acid, Omega-6 fatty acid and also palmitoleic acid. The oleic acid in macadamia nut oil has anti-inflammatory properties that makes it effective in fighting against chronic diseases, such as heart disease.

Macadamia nut oil is a stable oil that is also great for topical use for all skin types. I love macadamia oil for use on dry and mature skin due to its high concentration of palmitoleic acid. This acid is naturally present in human sebum when we are young and declines as we age; it softens and moisturizes the skin and also helps in healing mild wounds. Macadamia oil is absorbed very easily by the skin and the scalp and helps the cells to rejuvenate. It prevents sunburns and also helps the skin retain its moisture.

It also acts as an antioxidant. It prevents damage to skin cells by free radicals that cause signs of aging on the skin. Macadamia nut oil skin care is also attributed to its high vitamin E content. Macadamia oil is also a rich source of calcium, vitamin B complex and minerals like phosphorus and iron. Macadamia nut oil is VERY tasty for salads; it has a natural "nutty" flavor.

IN SUMMARY

One of the biggest myths about losing weight is that cutting out or limiting all fats is essential, when in reality eating healthy fats is a key part to losing weight and maintaining optimal health. There is a bit of truth in this myth in that completely cutting out "trans" fat from the diet is an essential part of losing weight and for reaching or maintaining the best health. But as for natural fats, they not only taste great, but are healthy. Previous studies had found that **97 percent, of the world's hunter-gatherer societies would have exceeded recommended guidelines for fat, yet they had no issues with the health problems we are having today.** Also, real weight gain is a pretty slow process. If you eat a very fatty meal and the scales are saying you've gained a few pounds, it's highly likely this is due to fluid. If you hang in there, and get back to eating healthy again, those few extra pounds will resolve themselves.

I want to start this section by reminding you that I am a former fat kid and I will always LOVE food. Before you read this and get depressed I want you to know that I still enjoy a dessert everyday…no lie. I just make them with things from my "Alternative Flour" section of this book and the "Alternative Sweeteners."

We all know that sugar is bad, but we mistakenly believe complex carbohydrates are healthy and we need to eat them in abundance. BUT what if I told you that complex carbohydrates are just glucose molecules hooked together in long chains. The digestive track breaks it down into glucose (sugar). So a sugary and a starchy diet are pretty much the same thing. When I write about sugar, I am also referring to starch.

Sugar is so gratifying. That first bite of heaven can calm us down and give us energy at the same time. It's like magic, with the power to flip our mood 180 degrees. That's the upside of sweets. The downside is that the more you eat them, the more you want them. Excess sugar causes a hormonal imbalance, which leads to carbohydrate cravings and weight gain, literally turning your body into a fat-making, fat-storing machine. However, I've got good news for you. You are in charge and can get off the fast track to diabetes; and you can do it naturally. An overconsumption of fat-free foods and a sedentary life can lead to a condition called insulin resistance; which is a physical imbalance that makes the body respond abnormally to carbohydrate-rich foods and causes people to gain weight.

Sugars are the simplest form of carbohydrate; which can be natural such as lactose (milk sugar) and fructose (fruit sugar), or can be refined such as sucrose (table sugar). All starchy foods, like potatoes, and sweet foods, like fruits, raise blood sugar quickly. When digested they are immediately absorbed into the bloodstream, causing an increase in the hormone insulin. Insulin clears sugar and fat from the blood and to be stored in the tissues for future use. This causes weight gain.

No matter where the carbohydrates come from; 4 grams of carbohydrates equal one teaspoon of sugar in our body. Let me say that again…4 grams of carbohydrates equal 1 teaspoon of sugar in our body. So with that thought, a small Blizzard has 530 calories and 83 grams of carbohydrates; which equals 21 teaspoons of sugar. A nine ounce bag of potato chips equals 32 teaspoons of sugar…add a soda, that's another 16 teaspoons of sugar.

1890 the average person consumed 2 teaspoons of sugar and in 2008 the average person consumed 56 teaspoons of sugar. WOW! This added sugar is mostly in the form of refined, white sugar. It is high in calories and devoid of nutrients. Extra sugar is being added to prepackaged foods. A piece of bread now contains refined sugar. Chocolate cake and other sweet delights can contain as much as 25 teaspoons of refined sugar, and that's not including the refined flour turning into sugar in our bloodstream! It's not just white sugar that needs to be consumed in moderation; brown sugar, powdered sugar, honey, and maple syrup are all sources of refined sugar. Eating too much sugar is part of an addictive cycle. When you eat sugar, it's quickly digested and burned, and it causes peaks and valleys in your energy level that leaves you craving more.

It is a dangerous situation when uninformed medical professionals recommend a high complex-carbohydrate, low-saturated-fat diet. A high complex-carbohydrate diet is nothing more

The food industry is responsible for a detrimental lie: that processed food, imitation food, is just as good as real food. Just because the "food" takes away our hunger pains, doesn't mean it nourishes our bodies to make them run properly. There are billions of dollars being made selling that "food." But to make that money, you have to spin things so that people don't really know enough to question their behavior. Advertising geniuses know that if you keep on repeating a lie, you end up with a lot of people believing it; I hate that the Dairy Council claims that low-fat dairy aids in weight loss…did you know there is a lawsuit about that claim now? The medical profession even bought into the industry's myths about cholesterol and fat; then they started pushing low-fat diets into the population without really investigating the science. That helped the food industry put all of these artificially created trans-fats into the food supply. And the more of that that went into the food supply, the fatter people became and the more they thought they needed to only consume low-fat foods.

than a high-glucose diet, or a high-sugar diet.

Your body's primary way of getting rid of sugar, because it is toxic, is to burn it with exercise. The sugar which your body can't burn will be stored as glycogen, and when our glycogen reserves are full, sugar gets stored as fat. Another major effect of insulin on fat is it prevents you from burning it. If you eat sugar your body will burn that instead of extra fat.

In the body, insulin has a very important job; it is secreted in response to elevated blood sugar levels, such as those that occur after a meal, and it pushes that sugar into storage. First to be filled are the tissues of the muscles and the liver where the sugar, which fat-free meals are filled with, is converted to glycogen. Glycogen is the body's fuel of choice for high intensity aerobic activity because it is readily available and because it is quickly converted to ATP for energy.

The problem is that the body only has storage for about 2,500 calories worth of glycogen providing your stores were totally empty, which is impossible. Most people only have room to store about 500 calories of glycogen from any given meal. After these storage areas become full, insulin pushes the left over sugar into the other unlimited storage area, FAT STORAGE.

The critical thing is not whether a food has sugar, but how quickly the sugar enters the blood stream. Food is actually categorized by this rate of entry. This is known as the glycemic index.

Insulin works hard at helping your body preserve energy from food and it does this in three ways. First, insulin tells your body to eat, particularly sugar or carbohydrates. If you follow those cravings, insulin rewards you by causing you to experience extreme gratification. Second, insulin escorts the energy from these foods, which is now blood sugar, to wherever it is needed in the body. It tells the liver to turn any extra energy into blood fat, triglycerides, to be stored in the fat cells. And third, it orders the body to keep the food energy locked inside the fat cells, not burning it for energy, but storing it up for a time in case of a famine.

Under ideal conditions, this insulin blood sugar regulation mechanism works perfectly in our bodies. When you're a kid and you eat candy loaded with sugar, your blood sugar increases and your pancreas releases a little insulin, which drives your blood sugar back down rapidly. The pancreas only releases a small amount of insulin because in children the cells are very sensitive to this hormone. This delicate sensitivity causes insulin to easily handle extreme amounts of sugar and carbohydrates that kids gorge themselves with, but not without a price. We may think it is fine for our kids to enjoy the simple pleasures of junk food, but they eventually develop a loss of sensitivity in the sensors to insulin, a condition known as insulin resistance.

This begins a cruel cycle of needing more insulin to keep the system going. As the body releases more insulin in an attempt to push through the resistance and force the precious blood sugar to the muscles and liver that need it, the extra insulin leads to carbohydrate cravings. In an attempt to calm our desire for carbohydrate-filled foods, even more insulin is released and to protect itself from too much insulin the body becomes even more insulin resistant. Eventually, the fat cells will shut down while the insulin gets stuck in the bloodstream which leads to adult-onset diabetes. As the years go by of overconsumption of refined carbohydrates and sugar, our bodies require higher levels of insulin in order to metabolize food appropriately and keep our blood sugar in the normal range.

The more sugar we eat, the more we crave it. If you start your day off with cereal and skim milk, you aren't going to be able to walk by the candy jar in your office at 2pm! Check out these to breakfast comparisons:

Option 1 = 1 cup SMART START Cereal (1 cup skim milk and banana)
    472 calories, 105 carbs, 4g fiber = 25.25 tsp of sugar in blood
    (IF you didn't add any sugar!)

Option 2 = 2 eggs, with 2 cups of mushrooms, peppers, onions
    190 calories, 9 carbs, 3 fiber = 1.5 tsp of sugar in blood

Option 3 = My homemade donut made with coconut flour
    217 calories, 7.4 carbs, 4.6g fiber = 0.7 tsp of sugar in blood!

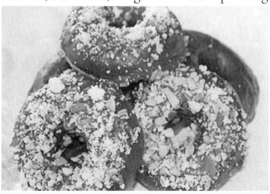

The human body evolved with a limited capacity to break down sugar, and in the past there was very limited access to it in concentrated forms, so processing the giant loads we consume today puts a huge strain on our bodies. Excess sugar lingers in the blood and causes trouble by attaching onto protein molecules, an age-accelerating process called glycosylation that causes cellular aging in several ways. First, it slows down the body's repair mechanism. Although glycosylation's effects are mostly internal, aging skin is a prime external sign. When excess sugar in the blood causes glycosylation, the skin loses its natural repair abilities. Sugar molecules clog up the collagen in your skin, which makes it less elastic, makes it wrinkle faster, and it can't heal as quickly if it's damaged.

Glycosylation also ages the body by spawning oxidative stress. Sugar molecules cut and irritate everything they touch, like shards of glass. The damage, called oxidation, eventually leads to a buildup of toxins. Eating poorly is like hitting the fast-forward button on aging. That's because, as toxins build up in the body, it damages the cellular engines called the mitochondria. I will talk about the importance of mitochondria throughout this book. It is responsible for so many things; not to mention it is what burns our fat! If we lose our valuable mitochondria we start having issues with weight, memory, hearing, vision and stamina. Cataracts can be due to glycosylation. Even more troubling are new findings that show

Other Names for Sugar:
Brown sugar
Agave
Corn syrup
Dextrose
Fructose
Fruit-juice concentrate
Glucose
High-fructose corn syrup (HFCS)
Honey: The honey bear is the only animal found in nature with a problem with tooth-decay (honey decays teeth faster than table sugar). Honey = highest calorie content of all sugars with 65 calories/TBS, compared to the 48 calories/TBS found in table sugar.
Invert sugar
Lactose
Malt syrup
Maltose
Molasses
Raw sugar
Sucrose
Syrup (Sorry Dad...maple syrup too)

overconsumption of sugar is linked to a piling up of arterial plaque in people with heart disease as well as in the brains of those with Alzheimer's and Parkinson's.

There are few people who can resist the taste of sweet foods. Food companies know this about humans, so they add it to their products to get us hooked on their brand. Major sources of sugar are sweets and candies, cakes and cookies, and fruit drinks, but they are also hidden in a lot of so called healthy food. **Healthy Choice frozen dinners can have up to the equivalent amount of sugar as 3 Snickers bars! And Fat-Free Yoplait yogurt has more sugar than a Kit Kat…I'd rather have the candy.**

PROBLEMS WITH TOO MUCH SUGAR:

1. High levels of insulin cause several problems: one of them is **high blood pressure.** One of the roles of insulin is to assist the storing of excess nutrients. Insulin plays a role in storing magnesium. But if your cells become resistant to insulin, you can't store magnesium so you lose it through urination. Intra-cellular magnesium relaxes muscles. What happens when you can't store magnesium because the cell is resistant? You lose magnesium and your blood vessels constrict. This causes an increase in blood pressure.

2. Insulin also causes the retention of sodium, which causes fluid retention, which causes **high blood pressure and congestive heart failure.**

3. A recent study showed that overweight children with high levels of insulin in their blood are also likely to have high levels of homocysteine, a substance which appears to raise the risk of **heart disease, stroke, and birth defects.**

4. **Osteoporosis** is another potential problem resulting from insulin resistance. Insulin is a master hormone which controls many anabolic hormones such as growth hormone, testosterone, and progesterone. In insulin resistance, the anabolic process is reduced. Bone is built upon the command of such hormones. When these hormones are reduced, the amount of bone building is reduced, and the amount of calcium excreted is increased.

5. Insulin increases cellular proliferation, which increases **risk of cancer.** Some pretty concrete studies show that one of the strongest correlations to breast and colon cancers are levels of insulin.

Fructose and Metabolism

Have you looked at the ingredients in your BBQ sauce? The first ingredient is usually corn syrup NOT tomatoes! But maybe you are saying, "I always make my own already." BUT how are you making it? My mom still uses ketchup...and what is ketchup? Nothing but gooey-red corn syrup.

You may be thinking, "Well, I don't buy the ketchup with high fructose corn syrup, I get the organic agave sweetened brands at health food stores." (such as the "organic" ketchup in the photo), but that is no better.

Agave Syrup is marketed as "low glycemic" and that is true, but let's look into why agave syrup is "low glycemic." It is due to the shockingly high concentration of fructose. It is 90% fructose and 10% glucose. Sugar is about 50/50% fructose to glucose, honey is about 55% fructose, high fructose corn syrup can range from 55-65% fructose.

WHY FRUCTOSE IS SO HARMFUL

1. Fructose can only be metabolized by the liver; glucose on the other hand can be metabolized by every cell in the body. Fructose raises triglycerides (blood fats) like no other food. Fructose bypasses the enzyme phosphofructokinase, which is the rate-limiting enzyme for glucose metabolism. Fructose is shunted past the sugar-regulating pathways and into the fat-formation pathway. The liver converts this fructose to fat, which, unfortunately, remains in the liver which equals FATTY LIVER DISEASE. **Consuming fructose is essentially consuming fat!** This is why I see so many children with fatty liver disease...they aren't drinking alcohol, they are drinking sodas, juices and consuming too much fructose!

2. Fructose **reduces the sensitivity of insulin receptors**, which causes type II diabetes. Insulin receptors are the way glucose enters a cell to be metabolized. Our cells become resistant to the effects of insulin and as a

result, the body needs to make more insulin to handle the same amount of glucose. We also start to produce insulin as a defense mechanism even if we don't eat and sugar or starch. YIKES! This is why we should allow our children to eat so much sugar and starch either...even though they are thin and active, you are setting them up for an adulthood where they can't enjoy a dessert without reaping the adverse effects. I grew up on Fruity Pebbles and skim milk for breakfast, Cocoa Pebbles for dinner, which is why I am so sensitive to glucose.

3. Fructose is high in uric acid, which **increases blood pressure** and causes gout.

4. Fructose increases lactic acid in the blood. High levels cause **metabolic acidosis** especially for those with conditions such as diabetes.

5. Fructose accelerates oxidative damage and **increases aging**. Fructose changes the collagen of our skin making it prone to wrinkles.

6. High consumption of fructose leads to mineral losses: iron, calcium magnesium and zinc, which can lead to low bone density (osteoporosis). It also interferes with copper metabolism. This causes collagen and elastin being unable to form, which are connective tissue that hold the body together. A deficiency in copper can also lead to infertility, bone loss, anemia, defects of the arteries, infertility, high cholesterol levels, heart attacks and inability to control blood sugar.

7. Fructose has no effect on our hunger hormone ghrelin and interferes with brain's communication with leptin, which is the hormone that tells us to stop eating and you can become leptin resistant! (see chapter on HORMONES for charts What to Eat.)

In June of 2009, I appeared on a television show called Twin Cities Live in Minneapolis, MN. I frequently did little cooking bits for optimizing our health. During one particular show, I made ketchup, BBQ sauce and marinara sauce. These are 3 sauces I always make because the pre-made versions are filled with high fructose corn-syrup. My favorite one is the Prego marketing genius that wrote "HEART SMART" across the front of the jar. This jar contained 10 extra grams of sugar per serving, and the serving size was tiny. Anyway, my point is that we add way too much cheap fillers like high fructose corn-syrup to food items. I started the television segment by explaining I had one client lose 15 pounds just by cutting out sugar in his condiments. He still enjoyed ketchup, just not the traditional kind. The night after the show I received this letter in my email...

LETTER FROM CORN COUNCIL PRESIDENT:

June 23, 2009
Maria Emmerich
Inspiring Actions
1810 Webster Street
Suite 5
Hudson, WI 54016

Dear Ms. Emmerich:

We viewed your June 22 appearance on "Twin Cities Live," with interest. There is a lot of confusion about high fructose corn syrup. We would like to provide you with science-based information on this safe sweetener.

High fructose corn syrup is simply a kind of corn sugar. It has the same number of calories as sugar and is handled similarly by the body.

The American Medical Association recently concluded that "high fructose syrup does not appear to contribute to obesity more than other caloric sweeteners." (American Medical Association. June 17, 2008. Press Release: AMA finds high fructose syrup unlikely to be more harmful to health than other caloric sweeteners http://www.sweetsurprise.com/sites/default/files/AMARelease6-17-08.pdf)

The American Dietetic Association concluded that "No persuasive evidence supports the claim that high fructose corn syrup is a unique contributor to obesity." (Hot Topics, "High Fructose Corn Syrup." December 2008. http://www.eatright.org/cps/rde/xchg/ada/hs.xsl/nutrition_19399_ENU_HTM L.htm)

High fructose corn syrup is used in the food supply because of its many functional benefits. For example, it keeps food fresh, retains moisture in bran cereals, helps keep breakfast and energy bars moist, maintains consistent flavors in beverages and keeps ingredients evenly dispersed in condiments. High fructose corn syrup enhances spice and fruit flavors in yogurts and marinades. In salad dressings and spaghetti sauce, it improves flavor by reducing tartness. In addition to its excellent browning characteristics for breads and baked goods, it is a highly fermentable nutritive sweetener and prolongs product freshness.

To read the latest research and learn more about high fructose corn syrup, please visit www.SweetSurprise.com. Please feel free to contact me if you would like additional information about the products made from corn.

Thank you for your consideration,

Audrae Erickson
President
Corn Refiners Association
Washington, DC
(202) 331-1634

MY RESPONSE:

Hello Audrae,

It is an undisputed fact among nutritional experts that we must reduce the amounts of sugar (HFCS, Sucrose, etc.) in our diet and that these sugars are the leading cause of our obesity/diabetes/etc. epidemic in America (See attached graph).

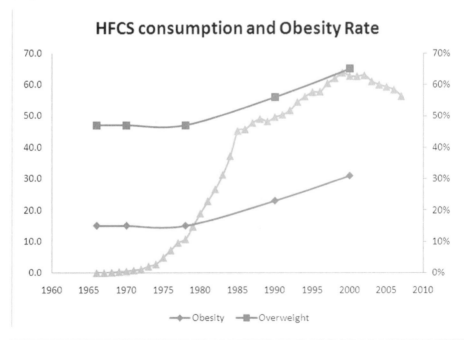

HFCS is one of the cheapest sweeteners due largely to farm subsidies. It is then used in a wide array of products due to its low cost. You prove my point here when you state the following products: "bran cereals, breakfast and energy bars , beverages condiments, spice and fruit flavors in yogurts and marinades, salad dressings and spaghetti sauce, breads and baked goods."

HFCS doesn't NEED to be in any of those products and shouldn't be. It's in children's vitamins and baby formula! HFCS (and corn syrup, corn syrup solids, and the other derivatives) is in nearly all processed foods (the foods that account for about 75% of the American diet).

The government spend billions of dollars subsidizing corn (below are totals for 05 and 06) which makes corn syrup so cheap that it is used in nearly every product. So we are spending billions of dollars to put something in our food that every nutritional expert says we need to eat MUCH less of.

Annual Government Corn Subsidies

005		$9,399,338,468
006		$4,920,813,719

So yes, I think that HFCS is the problem. Without it and the huge subsidies that make it so cheap, it wouldn't be in every food product on our grocery shelves and it wouldn't have created the problem we have today with obesity and diabetes, etc. Imagine if we spent all of those billions of dollars subsidizing broccoli and cauliflower production and it became one of the cheapest food options. Our country would have almost no problems with obesity.

You may also want to read this article:
http://www.westonaprice.org/modernfood/highfructose.html

Regards,
Maria

The next time purchase your favorite marinara sauce or open up your can of mid-afternoon energy boost of Mountain Dew, look at the ingredients. One of the first ingredients is high fructose corn syrup. People eat more sweeteners made from corn than from sugar cane, consuming it in frozen foods and baked goods without even knowing it. Did you know that Smucker's pancake syrup that tastes like maple syrup is nothing more than flavored corn syrup? The amount of syrup most people use on their pancakes can equal 500 calories…about the amount of calories I get in my whole breakfast of eggs with cheese and chicken sausage! But people think, "the syrup is fat-free," yep, all the more reason you have an insulin spike, store extra fat, and are hungry soon after.

Nutritional experts agree that high fructose corn syrup is a major culprit in this nation's obesity crisis. This government subsidized sweetener flooded the American food supply in the early 1980's, just about the same time the nation's obesity rate started to climb.

You may ask "Why does high fructose corn syrup make us gain weight?" Is it because of the overconsumption of Big Gulps? Or does the fructose in the corn syrups do something to our metabolism? The truth is that high fructose corn syrup is loaded with calories. A 12-ounce can of soda contains up to 13 teaspoons of sugar in the form of high fructose corn syrup. The average person drinks about *56 gallons* of soda in a year, or about three cans per day. That's 39 teaspoons of sugar; **our bodies only need one teaspoon of sugar per day to function!**

Even more interesting is that high fructose corn syrup is processed by the body differently than table sugar. It encourages the liver to dump more fat into our blood stream, fat that eventually ends up in our bellies. In the end, we are left still hungry soon after eating this junk, while storing more and more fat. High fructose corn syrup has been found to alter the function of hormones that regulate metabolism and cause abnormal weight gain.

Now that the FDA has officially changed its course and claim

When you eat real food, your body eventually releases hormones to help you feel satisfied. But fructose in high fructose corn syrup and agave isn't recognized by our brain as real food and never releases a hormonal signal of satisfaction. Your body wants you to keep eating so it can receive the nutrients it needs; which is why low-fat foods that replace fats with HFCS are extremely unhelpful with satisfying

Americans consume 450 calories a day from beverages, about twice as many calories as 30 years ago. These extra calories are so detrimental to our waist line…it amounts to gaining 23 pounds a year!

that High Fructose Corn Syrup does indeed qualify that it "would not object to the use of the term 'natural' on a product containing the HFCS produced by a manufacturing process without synthetic fixatives ," the corn refiners association is joyfully proclaiming its "naturalness" every chance they can find. They just launched a $30 million advertising campaign to place HFCS on the same level as sugar and honey. You can't miss the new commercials that claim false guidance as "it's made from corn and it's natural" while at the same time calling those who are concerned about the documented scientifically-sound negative health effects of high fructose corn syrup as uninformed worry-worts.

The commercials fail to let you in on what high fructose corn syrup can really do to our bodies. Let's take a look at what scientists, researchers and nutritionists (not the food producers who have an interest in making money) say:

1. High fructose corn syrup = cognitive impairment.
2. High Fructose Corn Syrup = high cholesterol.
3. High Fructose Corn Syrup = mineral imbalance = osteoporosis.
4. High Fructose Corn Syrup over-stimulates insulin = obesity.
5. High fructose corn syrup = non-alcoholic fatty liver disease.
6. High Fructose Corn Syrup and fructose = diabetes.
7. High Fructose Corn Syrup and fructose = atherosclerosis.
8. High Fructose Corn Syrup = metabolic syndrome.
9. High fructose corn syrup = kidney disturbances and disease.
10. High Fructose Corn Syrup = gastro-intestinal distress.
11. High Fructose Corn Syrup consumption in conjunction with low intake of magnesium (fairly common) = insulin resistance and hypertension.

The truth is this just because it's made from corn doesn't make it healthy; ethanol is also made from corn but I don't see anyone trying to mix it into Mountain Dew. Fructose, found in fruit, has a place in the human diet as long as it's consumed in moderation. High Fructose Corn Syrup on the other hand is all but impossible to consume in moderation when we consider it's found in almost every packaged food available in the super market.

I recommend limiting your sugar intake to as close to 0 grams as possible. Unfortunately, this takes a lot of detective work; is not as simple as cutting out soda. Corn syrup has snuck into foods that you never thought would have it; just as the crazy letter I received listed. For example, that low-fat, flavored yogurt you think you can enjoy without guilt often contains 10 teaspoons of sugar from high-fructose corn syrup; this is not a good option if you are trying to lose weight. You will also find it in lunch meat, hot dog buns, English muffins and even baby formula...that's right they want our children to be addicted as soon as possible. It is hidden in so many foods. I encourage you to be smart consumers and read every label carefully. The pay-off is worth it; you will experience fewer aches and pains, better blood sugar levels, along with better memory and focus. Best of all, when you step on the scale, the needle will rest on a lower number.

FAT BURNING TIP:
While it is important to stay well hydrated to burn fat, drinking liquids while eating is counterproductive. Liquids dilute your digestive enzymes; which break down food. A small amount of liquid during meals is okay but drinking a lot of water, juice, alcohol, or soda can cause indigestion and acid reflux...beer is the main culprit with acid reflux! Whenever possible, it is best to drink fluids before and an hour after meals as this helps absorb nutrients and move bowels. Reducing the amount of salt is helpful in reducing the need to drink fluids with meals.

Alcohol...it's not just the calories!

     Successful weight loss is all about oxidizing or burning, more calories than you eat. The primary problem with all alcohol is that the calories add up so quickly. At seven calories per gram, alcohol is a very calorically dense liquid that does nothing good for our body, no matter what you read in magazines...your risk of heart disease is NOT going to go down if you drink alcohol. I really hate those claims!

     When people go on a diet, they often choose the "light" version of their favorite alcoholic beverages in order to save a few calories. However, that is only a small piece of the puzzle. Alcohol has extremely damaging effects that is way more complicated than calorie counting.

Cocktail	Calories
Long Island Iced Tea	780
Frozen Margarita	740
Margarita	490
Pina Colada	460
Mai Tai	350
Sangria	310
Martini	160-175
Mojito	150-220

     The American Journal of Clinical Nutrition discovered that **fat metabolism is reduced by as much as 73% after only two alcoholic beverages in a one hour time period. This scary fact shows that the primary effect of alcohol on the body is not so much how many calories we consume, but how it stops the body's ability to use your fat stores for energy.** Alcohol in the body is converted into a substance called acetate. Studies find that blood levels of acetate are 2.5 times higher than normal after only two drinks and this quick rise in blood acetate puts the brakes on fat burning.

     Unlike a car that uses one supply of fuel, the body is able to draw from carbohydrates, fats and proteins for energy. The source of fuel or energy is determined by its availability. Therefore, when your blood acetate levels increase, your body uses acetate instead of fat. To make matters worse, the more you drink the more you tend to eat; and unfortunately, drinking will make your liver work to convert the alcohol into acetate, which means that the foods you consume at this time will be converted into extra fat on your body.

     If that didn't sound bad enough; alcohol can also stimulate your appetite and decrease your testosterone levels for up to 24 hours after you finish drinking. Athletes make a huge mistake by lifting weights the morning before a night of drinking in order to "earn their calories." As you lift weights, you break down your muscle, as you rest you rebuild and get more muscle…BUT we need testosterone for this to happen. Therefore if you workout really hard Friday morning, binge drink Friday night, you wake up Saturday morning with a slower metabolism than you had on Friday!

Also, we all know that alcohol dehydrates us. In order for fat to be metabolized, it must first be released from the fat cell and then be transported by the bloodstream where it is pushed to the liver to be used as fuel. If you are dehydrated, the liver has to come to the aid of the kidneys and can't focus on its role of releasing fat.

ALCOHOL AND HORMONE LEVELS

Not only does alcohol put the brakes on fat burning, it's also one of the most efficient ways to slash your testosterone levels; women…we don't want this to happen either. Just a single event of serious drinking raises levels of the muscle-wasting stress hormone called cortisol and decreases the levels of testosterone for up to 24 hours. The damaging effects of alcohol on testosterone are made even worse when you exercise before drinking. Your muscles depend on hormones for repairing them.

Women, have you ever experienced hot flashes after a drink or two? Estrogen is also affected by alcohol. Biochemically, the higher your level of estrogen is, the more readily you absorb alcohol, but the slower you break it down. Additionally, alcohol increases estrogen levels. Women often experience 300% increase of estrogen levels only thirty minutes after a drink; enter HOT FLASHES. Most breast cancers are estrogen positive; therefore, it is no surprise to doctors that women who drink heavily have a higher risk of having breast cancer.

This is what is going on in MEN too…a "Beer Belly" is nothing more than an "Estrogen Belly" that many post-menopausal women suffer from! The decrease in testosterone and increase in estrogen is also why men often lose their ability to stay erect after a night of heavy drinking.

NUTRIENT DEFICIENCY

Alcohol is metabolized extremely fast by the body. Unlike foods, which require time for digestion, alcohol needs no digestion and is quickly absorbed...no thermic effect of food going on here! Alcohol gets VIP treatment in the body, being absorbed and metabolized before other nutrients. Too much alcohol in the blood can lead to a deficiency in Vitamins B1, B2 & B3, as well as magnesium and zinc. These nutrient deficiencies can eventually cause restless leg syndrome, weakening of the heart muscles, poor skin, arthritis, cravings for salty foods, increase in bruising and prostate gland disorder.

FATTY LIVER AND LIVER DISEASE

Though alcohol affects every organ of the body, it's most dramatic impact is upon the liver. The liver cells normally prefer fatty acids as fuel, and package excess fatty acids as triglycerides, which they then route to other tissues of the body. However, when alcohol is present, the liver cells are forced to first metabolize the alcohol, letting the fatty acids accumulate, sometimes in huge amounts. Alcohol metabolism permanently changes liver cell structure, which **impairs the liver's ability to metabolize fats. This explains why heavy drinkers tend to develop fatty livers.**

A liver clogged with fat causes liver cells to become less efficient at performing their necessary tasks, resulting in impairment of a person's nutritional health. Fatty liver is the first stage of liver deterioration in heavy drinkers, and interferes with the distribution of oxygen and nutrients to the liver's cells. If the condition persists long enough, the liver cells will die, forming fibrous scar tissue. Some liver cells can regenerate with good nutrition and abstinence, however in the last stage of deterioration, or cirrhosis, the damage to the liver cells is the least reversible.

DEMENTIA

Dr.Daniel Amen, psychiatrist, clinical neuroscientist and author of "Making a Good Brain Great," tells us that alcohol is one of the most common brain toxins. He discovered through brain imaging that alcohol clearly damages the brain. Four or more glasses of wine daily increase the risk of dementia. A recent study by Johns Hopkins University reported that even small amounts of alcohol consumed daily physically shrank the brain, which can damage memory and other abilities.

DEPRESSION/ANXIETY/INSOMNIA

Alcohol causes depression, anxiety and insomnia. Initially, alcohol may aid relaxation BUT it is the worst things you could do, for in the end it can actually increase the severity of the symptoms of stress, anxiety and depression. You end up having to consume ever higher and higher amounts of alcohol in order to sustain its effects and as a result excess alcohol can cause or intensify stress, anxiety and depression. Alcohol acts by mimicking the activity and function of the chemicals already present in the brain that help us to relax.

Alcohol binds to GABA receptors in the brain which are our tranquilizing brain chemicals that reduce anxiety. When you consume alcohol it competes with the natural chemicals that are destined to bind with the GABA receptors, often flooding them causing a decrease in sensitivity which makes a decrease in peptide secretion. The physiological effects resulting from substance abuse are reversible but it can be a very slow process before the receptors return to a proper sensitivity level. Another way in which alcohol increases anxiety is because it increases lactic acid, which is an underlying factor in anxiety and panic attacks.

In the short term, alcohol can boost our serotonin but in the long term excess can actually lower these levels. **Forty-five minutes after drinking, whole blood serotonin concentration was significantly reduced.** Excess alcohol can cause depression because it interferes with the amino acid tryptophan which the body needs to produce the mood enhancing chemical called serotonin. Low serotonin causes extreme sleep disturbances.

IN SUMMARY

The key in developing a healthy body and brain is to make some sacrifices. Let's face it, eating and drinking are two of life's greatest pleasures. Some people are unwilling to give these up, but to me it isn't worth it. I would advise you not to drink at all. After giving up alcohol, I have found longer lasting pleasures that have no ill-side effects.

Fast food and our metabolism

In the Spring of 2011, Taco Bell was sued because their "taco meat" was only 35% beef; the rest was all fillers and preservatives. Everyone was grossed out by this fact, but what disturbed me even more was that if the "meat" was increased to be 40% the FDA approves the claim to call it "meat!" Now if that doesn't deter you from eating that junk, I don't know what will!

I didn't think I would enjoy the movie Supersize Me, but it was fantastic. I'm not one for documentaries, but Morgan Spurlock sure made this movie worthwhile! The first time at McDonald's he was offered to "supersize" his meal, Morgan Spurlock enthusiastically agreed; he had a rule that if he was offered a supersized meal, he had to say, "Yes." He received his meal and happily walked back to his car and gobbled down a giant burger, fries and soda. Before he even left the parking lot, he felt queasy, and his "not-so-happy meal" came back up. Even so, he continued to eat three meals a day at McDonald's as part of the 30 day experiment that became a hit documentary movie.

By the end of the month, he was 24 pounds heavier and his health was rapidly declining. His doctors frantically tried to get him to stop the experiment. Interestingly, he also was craving the same high trans-fat, high-sugar, high-carbohydrate meals that once made him sick. At the beginning of the movie, the food was clearly toxic to his system, but toward the end of the movie, he didn't feel right unless he was getting that same food in regular doses. He was irritable, anxious and depressed when he wasn't eating it because he was going through physical withdrawal. Large fast food chains spend a lot of money on scientists for food additives and smells that are addictive and sadly, it is working. Spurlock's case was so dramatic that nutrition experts use his movie to prove an important fact; not only is fast-food unhealthy, but it can also make you an addict.

The first thing that comes to mind when we hear physical addictions, we immediately think of alcohol, cigarettes and drugs. But research now shows that some of the ingredients in fast foods can have a similar addictive effect. Fast foods burgers, overstuffed burritos, French fries, soft drinks, milk shakes, and even "grilled" chicken breasts are loaded with sugar, highly processed carbohydrates, and over-heated oxidized trans-fats. And these are just the ingredients we know about.

Like thousands of other food additives in our nation's food supply, many of the flavor and texture enhancing ingredients in fast food have not been tested. The testing of brain damage is worked out for only a few ingredients, such as MSG and food dyes, which are toxins that stimulate the NMDA receptors in the brain. But a study published in 2005, showed obvious behavioral effects from food additives in fast food that indicate an addictive effect. The sugar, the trans-fat, the salt, the refined carbohydrates, and the physiological dependence is increased by the convenience, by the notion of a bargain, and by the marketing campaigns. You feel deprived if you don't get your fix.

One recent study found that caged rats overwhelmingly choose sugar sweetened water over cocaine when given the choice. Rat studies also have shown that eating high levels of trans-fat can cause the brain to secrete a chemical that encourages more eating and discourages physical activity and that one high trans-fat meal is enough to kick off this process. Sugar stirs up brain chemicals called beta-endorphin and dopamine, which are also activated by heroin and cocaine.

About half of all restaurant revenues in the United States are from fast food restaurants. People are attracted by the convenience, the price and the skillful marketing, much of it aimed at children. Once you're inside, it's hard to choose healthier options because smelling the sugar and fried foods entices pleasure chemicals in the brain. This spike in insulin and dopamine creates a euphoric feeling immediately after eating, but soon after, insulin levels crash, and mood plummets. Cravings for more sugar-filled, fried foods reload and the only cure for this feeling is to grab more harmful foods. So many times fast-food fans tend to overeat in order to feed their addiction.

Studies also show that overeating becomes habitual because they're not getting the nutrients needed, even though they consume enough calories in a single fast-food meal as should in a whole day to maintain their weight. Fast-food is extremely calorie-dense, but devoid of nutrients. Most of the products on the menu come from "food products," far removed from the farms, fields and orchards where food naturally comes from; which means they are less nutritious and our brain is never satisfied.

Burger King's Tender-Crisp chicken sandwich, large fries and large chocolate milk shake equals to be 2,340 calories. With this type of math, it's easy to understand how someone will gain weight. But more importantly it's the nature of those calories, and not the calories themselves. This lunch provides more than 10 grams of trans-fats, which causes our metabolisms to run very slowly…our bodies don't recognize this man-made fat.

One interesting study compared two groups of monkeys; one group consumed 8 percent of their daily calories from trans-fats and a control group that didn't eat trans-fats at all. The study focused on trans-fats and the impact on cardiovascular health, but the scientists were surprised to find another unpleasant effect…**the trans-fat group gained three times as much weight as the control group, even though both ate the same number of calories each day.** In addition, the weight was belly fat, which is a risk factor for diabetes and heart disease. The lesson is that we can't eat fast-food and then think we can just eat salad for the rest of the day to make up for the calories…the damage has already been done. I encourage my clients to create the food they crave at home; I even have a recipe for chili-cheese-fries. If you make the meal at home, without any tran-fats, even if it has the same number of calories, you are less likely to put on weight. Researchers found that frequent fast-food consumption was directly associated with changes in body weight and insulin resistance. In fact, it had a higher impact on health risks than a sedentary lifestyle or alcohol consumption.

AN AGE ACCELERATOR

Trans-fat is also an "aging accelerator." The gory details of its negative impacts could fill this book. Trans-fat is to chronic inflammation what gasoline is to fire. Inflammation ages you from the inside out by eating away at your telomeres, the caps protecting the ends of your chromosomes. Every time a chromosome divides, its telomere shortens. So telomere length is not only a sign of how old you are, but also a measure of how well your body is aging. Think of telomeres like the tips on the ends of your shoelaces; if they break the chromosomes fray. That's bad because the shorter the telomere, the less proficient the chromosome. If your telomeres are short, you lose your ability to restore your organs.

IS IT WORTH IT? We all know fast-food isn't ideal for our waist line, but here are some scary health issues to consider:
Acne: The boost of insulin after meal high in refined carbohydrates and sugar leads to a boost of sebum on the skin, which causes acne. Acne is a sign of skin inflammation caused by a "delayed food allergies." (see Food Allergy Chapter)
Fatigue: Most people feel great right after the boost in dopamine, but when your blood sugar crashes, your energy levels and your brain waves have trouble working efficiently.
Kidney Stones: The amount of sodium in fast food trumps any food item in the grocery store. Hospitals use to see one patient a month for kidney stones, but are now treating over 100 teenagers a week. This is directly linked to the overconsumption of fast food!
Cholesterol and High Blood Pressure: The over-heated, oxidized fats inflame and harden arteries; which is the cause of these detrimental health issues.
Constipation: Fast-food is low in fiber and slows down your digestive process and metabolism.
Flatulence and Leakage: In addition to a gassy effect, food intolerances to gluten, dairy and corn added to most items, can also lead to undesired secretions.
Toxic liver: Toxic chemicals in cheap meats and overly processed grains can hold back weight loss by disturbing the endocrine system, slowing metabolism, increasing inflammation and stress on the liver. (see Toxic Liver Chapter)
Bad Breath and Body Odor: Consuming new man-made chemicals in fast-food has been shown to produce undesired smells that spew out of your breath and sweat glands.

Trans-fat also adds years to your age by dampen chatter between cells. Cells need supple walls to talk to one another. The body makes cell walls out of fat; good fat equals healthy walls; bad fat equals patchy walls. Because trans-fat is man-made, the molecule has an unnatural shape. It's like forcing a square peg into a round hole; trans-fat's odd dimension speeds up aging.

Most fast food is filled with corn, wheat, soy and dairy because they are cheap government-subsidized fillers and are the main food allergens. Even the grilled chicken breasts are filled with carbohydrates. These ingredients cause water retention and inflammation because many people are sensitive to these common fast-food ingredients. Without knowing it, people suffer a "delayed food intolerance," which creates an inflammatory response in the body and causes high blood pressure, high cholesterol, fatigue and digestive problems.

Breaking a fast-food addiction is similar to breaking other addictions. It isn't easy, and once the habit is broken, cleansing the liver from all the toxins is extremely helpful in stopping the withdrawal. (See Toxic Liver chapter)

Milk: Does it really "Do a Body Good?"

This section is based on a question I receive almost daily by clients and friends; why do you recommend full-fat dairy? The truth is that low-fat dairy is overrated and full-fat dairy could have more going for it than you'd think. I also want to preface this chapter by mentioning that if you buy a jug of milk off the dairy cart in the grocery store, you aren't just drinking milk from one cow; one gulp of that white substance is from hundreds of different cows that have been pumped full of hormones…not so enticing anymore, is it?

So, you are in the grocery store and two jugs of milk sit side by side, one skim and one whole milk. Now, without any other information about the ingredients, which one has been scientifically proven to cause weight gain and heart disease, and which has been proven to support weight loss and coronary health?

If you're like most Americans you'll pick the skim milk as the healthier choice. And despite the fact that your answer would be marketed and advertised as the right choice, you'd be wrong.

We can thank the powerful food industry, not science, to the misinformation of low-fat dairy products and weight loss. In 2003 the National Dairy Council began assertively promoting the "3-a-day" marketing advertisement. They claimed that eating three servings of low-fat dairy products daily would contribute to weight loss, displaying photographs of thin celebrities like Jennifer Aniston in milk moustaches to get Americans hooked on this idea.

Not surprisingly, several large food manufacturers of cheese and yogurt also grabbed onto this brilliant marketing ploy, and soon the theory that low-fat dairy could aid weight loss became an unproven belief of Americans.

In 2007, this false advertisement of dairy's "three-a-day" weight-loss campaign was stopped after a lawsuit by the Physicians Concerned with Responsible Medicine. They charged that 24 of the 27 studies behind the claim had not only failed to prove a connection between dairy and weight loss, but they had all been studied by a single researcher and funded by the Dairy Council. The Federal Trade Commission ruled that the advertisements were false, and the Dairy Council was mandated to stop them.

But, those powerful images of skinny celebrities stick with us and have made a lasting impression. Most people have never heard of the lawsuit and it remains as extensively held belief among health professionals and Americans that fat will make you fat and low- to no-fat foods, especially low-fat dairy products, will give you a slender body like Jennifer Aniston.

The theory connecting low-fat dairy to weight loss was likely put together by the old popular misinformation of "lipid hypothesis." This theory that saturated fats cause heart disease and obesity was never proven. Despite a lack of scientific support, the hypothesis has been promoted by most food manufacturers since it was first proposed in the 1950s. In 1977, a Senate committee even published a low-fat proposal entitled "Dietary Goals for the United States" that marked the start of an industrial-food revolution that allowed manufacturers to endorse margarine and corn syrup as health foods! As the theory gained momentum, full-fat dairy products started being replaced and even became loathed by well-intended dietitians; in the meantime, low-fat dairy products stared to thrive.

Today, Americans buy almost three times more skim milk each year and half as much whole milk than they did in 1975. This would stun earlier generations of dairy farmers who cherished the richness of whole milk and often threw the skim to the pigs. Whole milk is now almost a dirty word. In 2008, Starbucks replaced its standard milk from whole to 2 percent, to portray the healthy adoption of the low-fat doctrine.

So here's the problem…during the same period that the consumption of low-fat fare rose in the United States, our rates of obesity, type 2 diabetes and heart disease multiplied exponentially! Health experts are attributing this to our replacing natural whole foods rich in nutrients, including naturally occurring fats, with nutrient-poor, processed foods filled with sugar, refined carbohydrates and man-made oils. This trend and a number of recent studies are finding that fats from whole foods, including saturated, are not the enemy we've been led to believe; and that low-fat dairy isn't the weight-loss ally it has been pushed as.

The Harvard School of Public Health have always insisted that evidence tying dietary fat and cholesterol to blood cholesterol and arterial damage are not the bad guys. The body produces cholesterol to heal inflammation and internal injuries; elevated cholesterol levels are in response to coronary damage not a cause of it. Harvard points out that a low-fat dietary approach can have a number of negative health effects, some of which are tied to reduced absorption of essential nutrients that can only be absorbed in the body when consumed with fats. People are at risk for deficiencies of the important fat-soluble vitamins and nutrients when they consume low-fat foods.

The Harvard study goes on to state that the popularity of a low-fat diets have caused "unintended health consequences" by encouraging increased consumption of refined carbohydrates and trans-fats. The bad press about naturally occurring saturated fats played a key role in encouraging people to embrace processed-food products like "I Can't Believe It's not Butter," powdered coffee creamers, and fake whipped-cream. These items are filled with trans-fats and carbohydrates; which were once praised as healthful replacements for foods containing saturated fats, but recent studies have proven them to be the true culprit to increasing obesity, diabetes and heart-disease.

An endocrinologist at Harvard, David Ludwig, MD, PhD, leads the distinguished OWL Program (Optimal Weight for Life) for childhood obesity at Boston University Hospital. He has had overwhelming success using a low-glycemic approach to weight loss rather than a low-fat one. Ludwig finds that too much insulin caused by high-glycemic foods are far more prone to cause weight gain than consumption of saturated fats;

including those in full-fat dairy products. Ludwig proves that fat helps restrain insulin levels and appetite.

No- or low-fat dairy actually functions as a hindrance to weight loss for people. When the fat is removed from milk, what remains are a significant amount of un-absorbable fat-soluble vitamins and a surplus of lactose, or milk sugar, with some protein but no fat to slow its entrance into the bloodstream; which causes a spike in insulin levels …remember …the fat-storing hormone! This doesn't even account for the plentiful amounts of sugar often added to low- and no-fat dairy products to make them taste palatable and improve their flavor in the absence of naturally satisfying fat I get so frustrated when I hear marketing "experts" recommend chocolate milk as a post-exercise recovery drink; yeah, if you are trying to put on weight!

It's also likely that if you do drink skim milk rather than whole you are going to consume a heck of a lot more; which is also true with low-fat yogurt, fat-free sour cream, low-fat ice cream instead of the real thing for three reasons:

1. It takes larger servings of low-fat foods than full-fat foods to stimulate hormones that switch on our bodies' satiety signals.
2. There's a psychological predisposition to feel that because we're "being healthy" by eating these low-fat products, we are justified to "make up for it" by eating more of them.
3. Low-fat foods don't keep us satisfied levels for as long because there's no fat to slow our insulin levels, which causes spikes and crashes in blood sugar, increasing cravings to desire more sugary carbohydrate-laden food.

As compared to full-fat dairy, low- and no-fat dairy delivers lots of fast-absorbing lactose, sugar, to the bloodstream; causing insulin spikes and results in sugar cravings. The amount of lactose decreases with every increase in milk-fat content. So skim milk has the most, where heavy cream has only trace amounts.

Not only does an extra dose of lactose potentially lead to insulin problems, many experts argue that most of us aren't genetically inclined to digest it well in the first place. Studies prove that about 70 percent of people are somewhat intolerant to dairy and lactose as adults. In fact, we stop producing lactase, the enzyme that breaks down lactose in the intestines, shortly after infancy, when we officially no longer need it. Consuming dairy may not make us instantly ill, but undigested lactose in the intestine can cause all kinds of undesirable issues, such as painful bloating, flatulence, diarrhea, stomach cramps, skin rashes, acne and ear aches. Think about it…we are the only mammals that continue to drink milk after infancy.

In the past, dairy-eating cultures consumed milk in its fermented state, from the unsweetened yogurt of the Middle East to the clabbered milk in South America. Soured dairy products like cheese and yogurt "predigests" the lactose during the production process; therefore it is well-tolerated. Fermentation promotes digestibility by effectively "predigesting" the lactose before it can cause trouble in the intestines. These cultures also consume the full-fat versions because they don't have food producers inventing fat-free dairy creations.

Also the suggestion of milk as a nutritional staple is foreign to most cultures. If they do consume fermented dairy, it is quite sparingly, not in an oversized glass several times a day. Dairy as a main source of nutrition is probably unwise for most of us. And for people who can't tolerate dairy, there's no reason to be worried about lack of dairy leading to nutritional deficiencies. Remember, Americans have the highest calcium intake, yet we have the highest rate of hip fractures.

> Research proves why our ancestors were right in embracing the fat and throwing the skim part to the pigs…pigs are fat right, yet they consume an overabundance of corn…no fat in that right? Oops, off on a tangent again! But, now that you understand why low-fat dairy is not all it's cracked up to be and has been oversold as a health food, but you are like my mother where a life without milk is too much self-denial, here are reasons to choose the naturally full-fat versions of dairy.

Metabolism

Science favors the consumption of some unrefined fats for kids trying to lose weight, because fats dynamically promote a steady metabolism. Fat is digested slowly, which helps decrease the rate at which carbohydrates are released into the system. This also makes the body more accessible to the hormone called glucagon which "unlocks" fat stores for energy. If there's too much insulin from eating high-glycemic foods; such as overly sweetened fat-free yogurt, the body stops glucagon production, which stops fat burning. Fat is also the nutrient that triggers the brain to feel satiety, which decreases overeating.

Fat-Soluble Vitamins

2 percent, 1 percent and skim milk, are required to be fortified with vitamins, but not whole milk, especially when it comes to vitamin A. That's because about 1,400 to 1,600 International Units (I.U.) are already in it. Skim milk has a slightly higher percentage of fortified vitamins D, E and K than whole milk, but it doesn't serve much purpose: All these vitamins are fat-soluble, so without fat, they pass out of the small intestine undigested.

Strong Immune System

Milk fat contains glycosphingolipids, which have been proven to have infection and disease fighting properties. Butterfat is an amazing fat; it has properties that maintain gut flora, it has nutrients that support your immune system, and it helps fight cancer. Vegetable oils and trans fats can't claim such amazing benefits.

Fertility and Sex Drive

The hormones that make us able to reproduce, testosterone, estrogen and progesterone, are created from the cholesterol produced by our bodies and is found in full-fat dietary sources such as milk and other animal fats. That's why statin medications used to lower cholesterol levels can also notably reduce sex drive. Eating full-fat dairy might also help women get pregnant; according to the Harvard School of Public Health, women who consumed at least one serving a day of full-fat dairy were 27 percent less likely to experience ovulation-related fertility issues.

So depending on you how much you enjoy dairy, if you can tolerate lactose, and it works with your biochemistry and metabolism are all things to consider if you chose to consume dairy or not; all of which are very individualized. The important thing is to recognize dairy's strengths and downsides. Choosing "Pasture-Fed" or "Grass-Fed" milk is a good first step. Pasture-fed cows have significantly more omega-3 fatty acids. It also contains a dietary compound called conjugated linoleic acid (CLA), shown to help reduce body fat and increase lean tissue (see CLA chapter). The key to the production of CLA appears to be in the fresh grass cows eat, so grain-fed dairy products won't have the same benefits. Pasture feeding is also the most humane method of keeping livestock, and the low-stress conditions keep stress hormones like cortisol and adrenaline out of the cow's milk. Also look for "USDA Organic," which guarantees that cows are getting organic-certified feed and aren't given antibiotics or bovine growth hormone (rBGH), which means the milk has fewer toxic byproducts. This is important for full-fat dairy, since toxins concentrate in fat.

Changing your mentality that we have a duty to chug 3 glasses of hormone filled milk a day and be free to discover different forms of dairy as a joy is step one. Step two is to understand that enjoying a creamy tasteful "umami" filled dollop of real cream is what life is all about.

In my family we use Almond Milk and Coconut Milk.

Unsweetened Almond Milk: It is extremely low in sugar and carbohydrates, and it taste great. It only has 40 calories per cup versus 90 calories for skim milk.

Coconut Milk: It is low in sugar and is healthy for SO many reasons...
1. DIABETICS: Improves insulin secretion and utilization of blood glucose. Helps relieve symptoms and reduce health risks associated with diabetes.
2. INTESTINAL DISORDERS: Helps relieve symptoms associated with gallbladder disease. Relieves symptoms associated with Crohn's disease, ulcerative colitis, and stomach ulcers. Improves digestion and bowel function. Relieves pain and irritation caused by hemorrhoids. Supports tissue healing and repair of the intestines. Improves digestion and absorption of other nutrients including vitamins, minerals, and amino acids. Reduces problems associated with malabsorption syndrome and cystic fibrosis.
3. ATHLETES: Provides ketones for a quick source energy. Boosts energy and endurance, enhancing physical and athletic performance. This also helps relieve symptoms associated with chronic fatigue syndrome.
4. IMMUNE SYSTEM: Kills viruses that cause influenza, herpes, measles, hepatitis C, SARS, AIDS, and other illnesses. It also kills bacteria that cause ulcers, throat infections, urinary tract infections, gum disease and cavities, pneumonia, and gonorrhea, and other diseases.
5. Kills fungi and yeasts that cause thrush, candida, ringworm, athlete's foot, diaper rash, and other infections.
6. Relieves stress on pancreas and enzyme systems of the body. Reduces symptoms associated with pancreatitis.
7. OSTEOPOROSIS: Improves calcium and magnesium absorption and supports the development of strong bones and teeth.
8. HEART DISEASE: Reduces inflammation. It is heart healthy; improves cholesterol ratio reducing risk of heart disease. Protects arteries from injury that causes atherosclerosis and thus protects against heart disease.

9. AGING: Helps to protect the body from harmful free radicals that promote premature aging and degenerative disease. Does not deplete the body's antioxidant reserves like other oils do. Improves utilization of essential fatty acids and protects them from oxidation. Prevents wrinkles, sagging skin, and age spots.

10. KIDNEY STONES: Helps protect against kidney disease and bladder infections. Dissolves kidney stones.

11. WEIGHT LOSS: It is lower in calories than all other fats and it supports thyroid function. It promotes weight loss by increasing metabolic rate. Is utilized by the body to produce energy in preference to being stored as body fat like other dietary fats. Medium chained triglycerides produce ketones (energy) rather than being stored as fat.

12. SKIN DISORDERS: Applied topically helps to form a chemical barrier on the skin to ward of infection. Reduces symptoms associated the psoriasis, eczema, and dermatitis. Supports the natural chemical balance of the skin. Softens skin and helps relieve dryness and flaking. Promotes healthy looking hair and complexion. Provides protection from damaging effects of ultraviolet radiation from the sun. Helps control dandruff.

13. Does not form harmful by-products when heated to normal cooking temperature like other vegetable oils.

Hemp Milk: Hemp milk is growing in popularity because of its flavor and texture. It also has lots of nutrients including calcium, tons of vitamins, minerals, and essential omega-3 and -6 fatty acids.

Meal plan examples

Here is an example of one of my client's "before" and "after" meal plans. This woman thought she was eating to lose weight, but in the end she realized she was way too hungry to sustain that diet plan. I feel this chart is quite eye opening. Her plan was filled with diet food, but it was also filled with too much sugar...no wonder why it didn't work!

BEFORE:

Time of Meal	Client's Food/Feeling	Calories	Sugar	Comments
7:30 a.m.	Coffee with Skim Milk…*hungry*	22	3	Skim milk has a lot of sugar (lactose)
8:00 a.m.	Multigrain Cheerios with Skim Milk and 8oz of grape juice… *Feel ok, not full*	470	64	High sugar, low protein food and no fat: this spikes your blood sugar and won't fuel a productive morning.
10:00 a.m.	A Banana… *Starving*	121	17	Another blood sugar spike, this will keep you hungry. Fructose spikes blood sugar faster than any other type of sugar.
12:40 p.m.	Slimfast shake… *Trying to eat "healthy"*	180	18	Slimfast contains too much sugar and you don't get the satisfaction of chewing.
1:15 p.m.	Yoplait Yogurt, Pineapple, and vitamin water	332	67	Blood sugar spike.
2:00 p.m.	Two pieces of hard candy	45	7	Another blood sugar spike.
3:00 p.m.	Diet Coke	0	0	
6:30 p.m.	Small salad with Fat-free French dressing, Spaghetti (1 cup) with marinara, and one piece of garlic bread	699	20	Too low in protein, no fat, and too many carbohydrates and sugar (marinara is notorious for added sugars)
9:45 p.m.	Fat free frozen Yogurt (1/2 cup)	100	18	Another blood sugar spike.

Even though this client consumed lots of food, she never felt satisfied, was often tired during the day and never felt calm…always on "edge."

AFTER:

Time of Meal	Client's Food/Feeling	Calories	Sugar	Client's Comments
7:00 a.m.	Coffee with real cream, 2 eggs with mushrooms and peppers and 2 slices of nitrate-free bacon...*Feeling kind of full but energized.*	289	0	Eaten within 1 hour of waking up. This meal is a good balance of proteins and healthy fats, thus it will hold her over for approximately 4 hours.
11:00 a.m.	Strawberry tea, Homemade Protein Muffin (my recipe) *Lots of energy and I'm in a good mood.*	195	3	Eaten 4 hours later, this is another fantastic protein-fat combo. She will be satisfied for 3 hours.
2:00 p.m.	Sandwich (Homemade Protein Bread), Turkey, Cheese, Lettuce, tomato and organic mayo) and ½ cup of Peanuts...*Delicious and I'm surprised that I'm not craving sugar.*	455	2	Eaten 3 hours after the last meal. She is sure to be burning fat and saving muscle because her blood sugar is stable.
6:00 p.m.	Caprese Salad, Chicken breast with alfredo sauce topped with mozzarella cheese, and garlic toast made with my Homemade Protein Bread... *This was good and I'm full!*	567	1	Eaten 4 hours later. She will continue to have stable blood sugar levels and feel great throughout the evening.
7:00 p.m.	No Sugar Added Ice Cream (1/2 Cup)... *A little desert to top off a great meal.*	90	4	A little desert if she wants right after the meal.

Now, the client had more energy, felt full and enjoyed the food more.

Meal Plan	Calories	Protein (g)	Carbs (g)	Sugar (g)	Sugar in Bloodstream (Teaspoons)
"Before"	1969	66	359	214	90
"After"	1696	138	30	10	10

CHAPTER 4

TYPICAL CLIENT PROBLEMS

The main problems I see with clients associated with weight gain are: Menopausal weight gain, Hidden Food Allergies, Tired Toxic Livers, and High Cholesterol diet mistakes.

Menopause and Weight Gain

Did you know… it takes your body 300 calories a day to ovulate? When our bodies stop ovulating, we stop burning an extra 300 calories per day. That equals to be 10 pounds per year!

So, what do we need to do to change that? The science of menopausal metabolism points to two major hormones, estrogen and progesterone. Many menopausal women have excess estrogen and a deficiency of progesterone. Our body produces 3 types of estrogen:

1. Ovaries produce healthy estrogen: Estradiol
2. Fat Cells store and form unhealthy estrogen: Estrone
3. 3rd type is produced only when pregnant: Estriol

Healthy estrogen from our ovaries gives women ample curves, attractive breasts and youthful skin. However, estrogen from our fat cells and external sources causes too many curves…or you might say 'bulges,' mainly in the belly area. Farmers have known this for years. They use a little synthetic estrogen to fatten their cattle. But women say to themselves:

"I don't take any form of estrogen. Why do I have too much?" The sad truth is that estrogen comes from our food choices. Our bodies make more estrogen when we eat too many processed carbohydrates. Insulin, the master hormone, is secreted from the pancreas in response to sugar and processed carbohydrates. Insulin stores fat and also causes our bodies to make more estrogen. This link to extra estrogen is also connected to Polycystic Ovarian Syndrome; which can cause fertility issues in young women.

Are you eating more fiber, taking the right probiotics, magnesium glycinate and still not going #2 everyday? Everyone should go #2 everyday...it is more important that you think. We are living in a sea of estrogens. When we aren't properly excreting those toxic levels of estrogens, they get stored in our fat cells which causes weight gain. Fat cells make estrogen and estrogen causes fatty tissue growth. This is a vicious cycle we'd like to avoid. Excess estrogen is excreted in the bowel. When stool remains in the bowel for a longer time, as in constipation, the estrogen is reabsorbed.

Some ways we get too much estrogen is exposure to chemicals that mimic estrogen such as many plastics (microwaving food in plastic dishes or using plastic wraps and containers) or eating non-organic food. Beef and chickens are typically given potent estrogenic substances ('super-estrogens') to make them more productive. Our produce is often laced with these substances.

People develop estrogen dominance as a result of a high-carb low-fiber diet, consuming excess fructose, drinking alcohol, having a "Tired-Toxic Liver (see chapter in Secrets to a Healthy Metabolism), or environmental factors...all of which we have some power to control. Even bar soaps leach estrogen's into our bloodstream.

The liver is a filter of sorts. It detoxifies our body, protecting us from the harmful effects of chemicals, elements in food, environmental toxins, and even natural products of our metabolism, including excess estrogen. Anything that impairs liver function or ties up the detoxifying function will result in excess estrogen levels. If your liver is tired and toxic, a special diet plan would be in order to help.

Estrogen is produced not only internally but also produced in reaction to chemicals and other substances in our food. When it is not broken down adequately, higher levels of estrogen build up. This is true for both men and women, although the effects are more easily recognized in men. Alcoholic men with impaired liver function develop a condition called gynecomastia, with estrogenic characteristics including enlarged breasts, loss of male pubic hair, and belly fat.

Some signs of excess estrogen in MEN and WOMEN:

- Migraines
- Low back pain
- Weight gain secondary to insulin resistance
- Belly Fat Accumulation (A "Beer Belly" is really an "Estrogen Belly")
- Fibrocystic breast disease
- Excessive PMS
- Menstrual disturbances--irregular and heavy bleeding
- Endometriosis
- Fibroids
- Ovarian cysts
- Breast Cancer

Correcting Estrogen Dominance involves more than just correcting the estrogen-progesterone balance and supporting the adrenals. It is important to eliminate the factors as much as possible. Exposure to xenoestrogens, insufficient sleep, toxic exposure, poor nutrition (high carbohydrates, low fat/protein intake, low nutrient value), and stress are some common causes. So, do you feel like you are eating the right way, taking the right supplements and STILL aren't going #2? It is most likely a food allergy!

FOODS TO AVOID AND FOODS TO EAT

The Special K cereal with a banana and glass of juice that once worked for breakfast is now too high in sugar and it creates an insulin response. Insulin produces more estrogen, which creates more fat cells, which make more estrogen that creates more fat cells. So, your waist size increases, and your clothes are too tight! At this time in life, you need to reduce the processed carbohydrates, which will reduce the amount of glucose in your blood. With balanced blood sugar levels, less insulin is needed and less body fat is created. For better metabolism at menopause, eat less cereal, pasta, bread and sodas. Instead, start eating more vegetables, healthy fats, and real protein.

Unless the meat you eat is labeled "no hormones added," you are probably eating meat with added hormones. Many commercial farmers of beef and sheep use hormones to promote rapid weight gain in their animals. The European Union has concluded that meat from animals fed hormones is bad for human health, but the US government has declared this practice safe. The best choice is organic, grass-fed meat which contains CLA (conjugated linoleic acid). Grass-fed animals have twice as much CLA as animals fed grains, and numerous studies have shown that CLA promotes healthy metabolism.

Peri-menopause and menopause are times when women need to pay attention to nutrition and food choices in order to maintain normal weight and a sense of well-being. Weight gain or mood swings might be the result of an insulin response or poor food choices, but there are other possible causes. Lack of sleep, too much stress, insufficient progesterone, adrenal exhaustion, and inflammation all may contribute to your menopausal issues. Interestingly, all these factors have a nutrition connection.

Food Allergies and Sensitivities

Do you have desires for a particular food and find it hard to satisfy your craving unless you eat that particular food? Have you ever eaten a bowl of cereal and almost felt hungrier than before? Do you have acne? Do you have eczema? Do you have bowel issues or stomach pain after eating? Are you depressed? Do you have a thyroid issue or other autoimmune disease?

If you notice these issues, then you probably have a food allergy. Another sign of a food allergy is carrying extra pounds no matter what you do. Around 11 million Americans suffer from food allergies. The eight major food allergens are: milk, eggs, peanuts, tree nuts, fish, shellfish, wheat and soy. In Oriental countries, rice is a prominent allergen. Among vegetables, white potatoes and lettuce are potent allergens. Scientists found that 92.2 percent of hospitalized schizophrenic patients were allergic to one or more common allergens; 88 percent of them were allergic to wheat, 60 percent to milk, and 50 percent to corn.

Once a food allergy exists, the food becomes mildly addictive and you can feel compelled to eat it. Food sensitivities may cause allergic people to crave those foods to which they are allergic. People with allergies experience uneasiness when they lose access to a particular food just as a drug addict suffers withdrawal symptoms when the drug is withdrawn. Food allergies will cause your body to react by storing it instead of using it for energy and weight gain will result. Compulsive cravings will also impede weight loss. The sad thing is that people with allergies have no idea that these daily food cravings and eating habits are based on a physiological need to control withdrawal symptoms caused by food allergy addiction.

There are two types of allergic reactions.

1. **Type A** (classic allergy). In this type of allergy, you experience a reaction immediately after contact with an allergen; such as shellfish or peanuts, and can cause swelling in the throat or more serious reactions.
2. **Type B** (delayed allergy or intolerance). The reactions from type B can take place one hour to 3 days after eating the food. Symptoms are weight gain, bloating, water retention, depression, fatigue, aching joints and headaches.

The phenomenon of allergies and addictions to both foods and chemicals is now well established by doctors specializing in the diagnosis and treatment of allergies. These doctors believe that many chronic health problems, such as migraines, fatigue, mood disorders, and arthritis are often caused by allergies to foods and involve around one-third of the people living in America. Food sensitivities and allergies have a huge effect on the portion of the brain that controls our emotions, memory and body functions, such as body temperature, hunger, thirst, sleep and blood pressure. It has recently been proven that 85 percent of migraine sufferers could be symptom-free when the followed a diet excluding the ten most common food allergens. The most problem-some allergens were cigarettes, coffee, and birth control pills. The studies also found that these allergens caused arthritis, asthma and diabetes.

Be aware that the same food can cause different reactions in people. A person's genetic disposition to allergies will determine which part of the body will become the vulnerable target. Any major organ may be affected: the symptoms of cerebral allergies are hyperactivity, ADHD, depression, irritability, headaches and some forms of schizophrenia; hypoglycemia is a sign of pancreatic malfunction.

Water retention is very common among people with allergies and is a contributing factor to obesity. When people go on an "elimination diet" to remove the offending food they will often lose five to ten pounds of water weight within a week. This initial water loss will help people lose fat more easily, even without dieting. Food sensitivities can cause the body to retain both water and fat.

People who are addicted to coffee do not necessarily get fat. People who are addicted to sugar or wheat, may end up running around with candy or wheat crackers to satisfy cravings. It's extremely difficult for people with allergies to lose weight unless they ultimately gain control of their food cravings. First off, it is hard to identify the specific allergen, and then they have to control the craving and then eliminate the food; which means lots of self-control.

The allergic reaction from a food can cause a drastic reduction in blood sugar followed by weakness, hunger and irritability. Allergic hunger does not respond to the satiety control center in the brain, so both the addictive and allergic responses can cause uncontrollable eating behaviors. For example, people who are allergic to sugar have an intense craving for sweets. One doctor had a patient who ate 30 Snicker's a day and although her stomach would hurt, she couldn't stop. When she was alone, she would sneak a tablespoon of sugar because it would make her feel good. She would actually get high on sugar, but it didn't last long. Three or four hours after eating she would go into a deep depression and even became suicidal. The withdrawal symptoms brought on the suicidal feelings. The woman's physician found her food allergy and she now reads all food labels for the trigger ingredients.

Adding vitamin C, calcium, magnesium and potassium can help neutralize the acidity caused by allergic reactions, ease stress, and inducing relief. This combination of nutrients, along with amino acid supplements, can totally knock out hunger cravings caused by food allergies as well as eliminate the withdrawal symptoms once the items have been eliminated.

If this combination eliminates your hunger then you can be sure that it was brought on by an allergy.

Many people make the mistake of running to their doctor for an allergy blood-test to find out if a food allergy is the root of their problems. The main issue with this is that blood tests are about 90 percent INACCURATE! Crazy, but true. If I notice a food sensitivity with a client, our success comes by an elimination diet along with nutrition therapy of enhancing vitamins, minerals and amino acids. It is also helpful to consult a doctor, but don't wait for a blood test to tell you what will make you feel your best...start now instead.

My suggestion is for everyone to cut out grains. I see so many people not have the afternoon lows, feelings of depression, water retention...you name it, they just feel better! Go to "Alternative Flours" chapter to learn more on how to satisfy your "bread cravings" without the wheat.

Tired toxic liver

Your liver plays a major role in weight loss. The liver is a chief organ in the body for metabolism functions. Keeping our liver at optimal health should be a main focus of your weight loss plan.

The liver makes and secretes bile for storage in the gallbladder. During digestion, the bile is moved to the intestine to break down fats. But, if the liver is congested, it doesn't produce enough bile for fat to be broken down. The liver can become congested from chemicals, toxins, drugs and heavy metals. Evidence of a "fatty liver" is often shown by a roll of fat at the waistline, which happens because the liver has stopped breaking down fat and started storing it. Only once you bring your liver back to full function, will you lose this fat.

Like every American, you're probably totally puzzled on which is the right weight loss plan. You've been flooded with emails of new miracle diets, and wondering if there are any health risks associated with them. Before choosing a weight loss programs, you need to discover if your liver could be to blame for your issues. When the liver is overloaded and toxic, every organ in a person's body is affected and weight loss efforts are stalled. Some signs of a toxic liver are weight gain, cellulite, abdominal bloating, indigestion, fatigue, mood swings, depression, high blood pressure, elevated cholesterol, and skin rashes. Many people struggle with weight gain and a sluggish metabolism most of their lives, and go through lots of yo-yo dieting unsuccessfully. "So why doesn't anything really work?" we may ask. We have been tackling the symptom when we should be addressing the cause; weight gain is often due to poor liver function.

The liver performs more than 400 different jobs, and is the body's most important metabolism-enhancing organ; it acts as a filter to clear the body of toxins, metabolize protein, control hormonal balance and enhance our immune system. Your liver is a "worker bee" that can even regenerate its own damaged cells! But our liver is not invincible. When it is abused and lacks essential nutrients, or when it is overwhelmed by toxins, it no longer performs as it should. Fat may build up in the liver and just under the skin, hormone imbalances can develop, and toxins increase and get into the blood stream.

The liver metabolizes not only fats, but proteins and carbohydrates for fuel. It breaks down amino acids from proteins into various pieces to help build muscle; which directly impacts your calorie burn. It also transports amino acids through the blood stream for hormone balance; which is critical to avoid water retention, bloating, cravings, as well other undesired weight issues. Amino acids also help move waste, such as damaged cholesterol, and used estrogen and insulin to the liver, for detoxification and elimination through the kidney.

The liver's most important function, and the one that puts it at greatest risk for damages, is to detoxify the numerous toxins that attack our bodies daily. Working together with the lungs, kidneys, skin and intestines, a healthy liver detoxifies many damaging substances and eliminates them without polluting the bloodstream.

When we cleanse the liver and eat the right foods, liver metabolism will improve and we start burning fat. As liver function improves, so does energy. With more energy, fitness improves, because we have the ability to exercise more and improve our muscle tone.

Cleansing the liver, not only will we shed excess pounds, we'll also lose some of that bumpy cellulite. Scientists discovered that cellulite is caused by inefficient removal of wastes from the body. As toxic materials collect between the cells, they are held by hardened connective tissue where they build up to create pockets of water, toxins, and fat that give the skin that unsightly bumpy appearance. Ridding the body of overly processed, prepackaged foods will help stop the accumulation of the lumps and bumps, and it will increase cell vitality.

The following are the most common symptoms of a toxic liver; being edgy, easily stressed, elevated cholesterol, skin irritation, depression, sleep difficulties, indigestion, kidney damage, heart damage, brain fog, hypothyroidism, chronic fatigue, weight gain, poor memory, PMS, blood sugar imbalances, allergies, or obesity. The liver also plays a role in migraines. If this vital organ is overloaded with toxic substances, it can cause inflammation that triggers migraine pain. If you have tried many ways to improve your health and energy level and nothing seemed to help, it is possible that your tired liver is triggering your difficulties. Restoring liver function is one of the most essential actions you could ever do for your health. When the liver gets congested it will remain that way and get worse until it gets cleaned and revitalized.

FOODS TO EAT

Every day, for at least one week, choose at least one serving from each group of the following liver-cleansing foods:
Cruciferous vegetables: cabbage, cauliflower, Brussels sprouts, broccoli
Green leafy vegetables and herbs: parsley, kale, watercress, chard, cilantro, escarole, dandelion and mustard greens
Citrus: lemons and limes (avoid grapefruit and grapefruit juice, which contain a compound called naringen that can get in the way of the liver detox). **Fruit contains fructose which is damaging to our liver, so stay to low sugar fruits, if any.**
Sulfur-rich foods: garlic, onions, eggs and daikon radish
Liver healers: artichoke, asparagus, celery, dandelion-root tea, and whey protein
Colon-cleansing foods: powdered psyllium husks, and ground flaxseeds.
Water: every day, drink half your body weight in ounces of water. Adding 1 tablespoon of UNSWEETENED lemon juice to your water can also aid in liver cleansing.
Protein: have at least two servings of protein in the form of lean beef, lamb, skinless chicken, turkey or fish, or, if you're a vegan or vegetarian, at least 2 tablespoons a day of a high-quality blue-green algae or a spirulina.
Omega 3's: 1000mg of a quality Krill Oil at each meal.

Are you consuming fruit for a snack or breakfast? Grabbing a banana for breakfast is a bad thing to do for your liver, yet so many people do this thinking it is helpful for weight loss. Fructose, the sugar in fruit is really hard on our liver. Think of fruit (and only the low-sugar berries) as an occasional treat. Agave should also be avoided since it is chemically 90% fructose (sugar is 50% fructose).

Our bodies are equipped with intricate systems to excrete toxins and waste through the skin, kidneys, lungs, liver and colon. But with exposure to trans-fats, food additives, synthetic personal care products, and chemicals in our water and air, the human body can become overloaded with too many chemicals to detox them efficiently.

There are many steps to help restore the vitality of your liver. Some liver stressors are caffeine, sugars, trans-fats, chocolate, soft drinks, many over the counter medications, cholesterol lowering drugs, anticonvulsants, and an inadequate intake of fiber. **Women detoxify caffeine slower than men because of hormonal interactions with caffeine. Birth control pills also increase the time to detox caffeine by twice as much.**

Sugar is also a terrible and very common liver stressor. You may say you don't consume sugar, but you may be ingesting it from a lot of prepared food quite unknowingly. Always read the labels; it is hidden in marinara sauce, ketchup, salad dressings, the list is scary. In the process of being metabolized, sugar robs your body of important nutrients; for example zinc, is essential for liver function. Sugar also restrains your liver's production of enzymes, needed in the detoxification process.

A major liver stressor is trans-fats like margarine. Trans-fat obstructs your liver's ability to burn fat. Our body will never learn how to process those "plastic-like" man-made fats.

Some medications also cause the liver to work harder. Sometimes it's best to look for a natural form of healing to replace a synthetic product. Coenzyme Q 10 is one way to help your cholesterol (see Supplement chapter). Always check with your physician first.

Not eating enough fiber also puts pressure on the liver. Fiber helps to remove toxins out of the body. Insoluble fiber absorbs water in the digestive tract and speeds up the time taken to move material and toxins out through the intestines. Without adequate fiber, 90% of cholesterol and bile acids will be reabsorbed and re-circulated to the liver. This taxes your liver and reduces its fat burning abilities.

Overwhelming evidence has proved that alcohol itself is toxic to the liver, even when nutrition is adequate. **Alcohol interferes with the liver's ability to metabolize hormones, which are important for maintaining blood pressure.** Having one drink can cause acute liver inflammation. As the liver breaks down alcohol, by-products are formed, such as acetaldehyde. Acetaldehyde is approximately 30 times more toxic than alcohol, and is a major cause of hangovers. Drinking alcohol depletes a store of a liver peptide called GHS, which helps us detoxify chemicals. Much of the cell damage that occurs in liver degeneration is believed to be caused by free radicals, highly reactive molecular fragments, liberated during alcohol metabolism. The damage caused by free radicals can include the destruction of essential components of cell membranes. Acetaldehyde appears to be the key generator of free radicals. Alcohol also stimulates the liver to make more triglycerides, and even a 2 oz. glass of wine a week can raise triglyceride levels. Stay Away!

TIPS FOR A HEALTHY LIVER

Fiber, fiber, fiber! It assists the liver by ridding the body of toxins. It is like a magic sponge that cleans our bodies.

Limit or cut alcohol completely.

Stop drinking soda, coffee, and caffeinated beverages. **In the long run, these only sabotage better health and a slimmer body.**

Don't eat white. Breads, white flour, and white sugar are bleached and heavily processed.

Don't starve yourself. Starvation dieting only slows down metabolism.

Go organic. Non-organic fruits & vegetables put more pesticides into your body.

Try adding more fresh lemons, virgin coconut oil, apple cider vinegar, to your diet, all of which promote healthy weight loss and cleansing.

Cut our gluten, found in wheat, rye, barley and all their related products, such as packaged cereals, macaroni and cheese, pizza dough, pasta, tortillas, pancake/waffle mixes and cookies, soups, as well as in many sauces, such as soy sauce.

Avoid soy protein isolates, found in many protein energy bars and processed soy foods

Replace **sugars** including agave, honey and maple syrup with **healthier sweeteners** like stevia, which balance blood sugar levels, support the pancreas, and do not promote weight gain.

Water (with a few tablespoons of UNSWEETENED lemon juice), turmeric and flaxseed act as antioxidants and provide nutritional support for liver detoxification pathways.

Red meat such as grass fed beef and lamb normalize liver enzymes in the blood.

Garlic and onion also aid in liver function.

Adding dandelion root can help cleanse the liver and aid in fat metabolism.

Switching to a natural make-up, deodorant and cleansing routine can also decrease the amount of toxins getting in through our porous skin.

Avoid over-the-counter drugs (use magnesium citrate for headaches instead)

Avoid Fructose: Agave is 90% fructose. The liver has to work to 80% capacity to work off fructose as compared to 20% to work off glucose.

Did you know that cholesterol levels are a very poor predictor of future heart attacks? The risk of future heart attacks has everything to do with excess levels of insulin. This is why diabetics are known to be at a high risk of heart disease.

Scientists used to think we had to worry only about our total cholesterol level, but then researchers found this wasn't a very strong predictor of heart disease. Next came the realization that there was both "good" (HDL) and "bad" (LDL) cholesterol. This launched a war against "bad" cholesterol, which is predominantly elevated by saturated fat.

We now know that there are 2 types of LDL cholesterol:

1. Large, fluffy LDL particles that appear to have no potential to cause atherosclerosis or the development of plaques on the large or medium-sized arteries.

2. Small, dense LDL particles that are strongly associated with arterial plaques and this can increase the risk of heart disease.

To determine which type of LDL = find your ratio of triglycerides to HDL

- If ratio is less than 2, you have fluffy LDL particles that are not going to do you much harm.
- If ratio is greater than 4, you have small-dense LDL particles that increase the development of atherosclerotic plaques – regardless of your total cholesterol levels.

Harvard Medical School has confirmed the importance of this ratio; the higher your TG/HDL ratio, the more likely you would be to have a heart attack. In some cases 16 times more likely!

Improve your TG/HDL ratio in 2 ways:

1. Lower your insulin levels. Excess insulin = increase triglyceride levels. Eat the "healthified" low carb way!
2. Supplement with high-dose, ultra refined-grade fish oils at every meal.

Cholesterol statins are also powerful anti-inflammatory agents, but not without consequences. They do lower C-reactive proteins; they worked like aspirin to reduce inflammation and therefore reduce heart attacks. Only statins cost a lot more and are less effective. The statins also include some serious side effects:

1. Muscle wasting = slower metabolism = higher triglycerides = snowball effect
2. Decrease cholesterol-production in brain = decreased production of new synaptic connections and loss of memory.

Has anyone noticed that the advice we've been given to cut out all foods high in saturated fat and cholesterol and embrace "I Can't Believe It's Not Butter," has actually increased our rate of heart-disease? These dietary changes have stopped us from benefitting from cholesterol's health-supporting roles in the body, robbed us of our pleasure in eating, increased obesity and resulted in widespread overmedication. It has also discouraged us from embracing a high-nutrition, anti-inflammatory diet and exercise to decrease risk of heart disease. Combining a low carb diet to control insulin with high-dose fish oil (to decrease inflammation) is the answer to decreasing risk of heart disease.

Over the past several years, as the role of inflammation in disease has become better understood, a growing number of well-recognized experts have begun agreeing that much of what we've been told or assumed was true about cholesterol is just plain wrong. Some awesome books to explain further are: "The Cholesterol Myths" by Uffe Ravnskov, MD, PhD; "The Cholesterol Hoax" by Sherry Rogers, MD; and "Know Your Fats" by biochemist Mary Enig, PhD.

After numerous studies, doctors and scientists are now finding that cholesterol in the diet is a minor player in heart disease. Scientific evidence points to high cholesterol as a sign of inflammation-based diseases like heart disease, rather than a root cause. Meanwhile, science is also revealing that trans-fats, sugars, refined carbohydrates are the main offenders in creating inflammation. So staying away from egg yolks, butter or prime rib aren't the problems in our diet; which means it's time for health-concerned people everywhere to reconsider what we thought we knew about cholesterol, and its true role in maximizing our health.

Myth No. 1: Cholesterol is bad for the body

Did you know that cholesterol is essential to many of our bodily functions? Cholesterol is a waxy white substance found in fat. It's one of a group of compounds called lipids and they are vital to the body's basic functions. It makes and repairs cell membranes, communicates between cells, absorbs vitamin D, and produce hormones; such as estrogen and testosterone. Lipoproteins are also part of our immune system, where they bind and neutralize bacteria, viruses and toxins.

A low level of cholesterol not only causes issues with our physical health, but also our emotion health; including depression. **Depression is caused by low cholesterol levels because it helps make serotonin; which is an important chemical in the brain that helps regulate our mood.** Low cholesterol levels are also a sign of serious illnesses; such as an overactive thyroid, liver disease, anemia, cancer and poor absorption of foods causing malnutrition.

The average person ingests between 200 and 300 milligrams (mg) of cholesterol a day from animal-derived foods, such as cheese, egg yolks and meat. But that's only a small portion of the body's normal cholesterol requirement; the average healthy person needs about 1,000mg a day. The liver makes up the difference, generating cholesterol from a variety of fats, proteins and carbohydrates available in the bloodstream.

"When we eat large amounts of cholesterol, our body's production goes down," writes Dr. Ravnskov in Fat and Cholesterol are GOOD for You!: What REALLY Causes Heart Disease. "When we eat small amounts, it goes up."

Our body regulates its cholesterol production; therefore, the amount of cholesterol in your blood is based on its needs for cholesterol. And one of the things that determine the body's level of need is the presence of free radicals, infection and inflammation. The more inflammation, oxidation or irritation present in the body, the more cholesterol the body produces in an effort to help tackle the problem.

"Cholesterol is much more of a good guy than a bad guy," writes Rogers in The Cholesterol Hoax. "Cholesterol is a messenger giving you a last-ditch warning." One shouldn't kill the messenger just because he brought you the message that you are in trouble." Not only is high LDL cholesterol not the cause of this arterial inflammation, it is actually the "brave fire-fighter" that, working with other lipoproteins, is an important helper in our immune system, heroically striving to put out the fire that has been started and repair damage already done.

The true problem lies with uncontrolled blood sugar, free-radical activity, toxins and other high inflammatory factors that inflame the arteries by creating tiny tears in the arterial walls. The body attempts to patch and heal the tears by putting down a thin layer of cholesterol, which acts like spackle or plaster. But if the root causes of arterial damage and inflammation go unaddressed, those well-intended cholesterol-composed plaques begin to add up and stiffen. Eventually, if irritated and inflamed, they can burst, blocking the arteries with debris and setting the stage for a heart attack.

The basic principal that I want you to take away is that, in the absence of inflammation, cholesterol is not the problem we once thought it was. Cholesterol is not the real enemy; inflammation is. And inflammation is not driven by dietary cholesterol or saturated fats, but rather by trans-fats, sugar, refined carbs, an inactive lifestyle and the presence of an infection in the body.

Myth No. 2: High blood cholesterol is caused by eating too much fat and cholesterol

I wrote a cookbook and I make individualized meal plans for my clients. They are often shocked to find the recipes using butter and red meat. The theory that there is a direct coloration between the amount of saturated fat and cholesterol in one's diet and the prevalence of coronary heart disease is known as the "lipid hypothesis."

As you read ahead, you will find that the old idea of cholesterol clogging the arteries is not true, and that when eaten in moderation with inflammation-reducing veggies, eggs and red meat shouldn't be off-limits to cholesterol-concerned people. Here are the things that influence our cholesterol:

1. **Trans-fatty acids:** These "bad-boys" are the root of many problems. They raise LDL and lower HDL and have a worse effect than saturated fats on the overall cholesterol ratio. That is why "I Can't Believe It's Not Butter" is a terrible replacement for butter.

2. **Monounsaturated and other healthy fats** (like those found in nuts, fish, olive oil and avocados) INCREASE the activity of LDL receptors in the liver and thereby lower LDL levels in the blood.
3. **Overeating and under-exercising** raise cholesterol levels by increasing abdominal fat stores. Abdominal fat also decreases insulin sensitivity, causing excess glucose to build-up in the bloodstream and intensify the formation of arterial plaques.
4. **B vitamins** (mainly folate) reduce blood levels of homocysteine, which assists in amino acid metabolism. Elevated homocysteine levels are an important risk factor for heart disease.
5. **Plant sterols and stanols** (the plant equivalents of cholesterol) reduce cholesterol levels by blocking cholesterol absorption, as well as dietary fiber.
6. **Antioxidants** reduce the oxidation of LDLs in the bloodstream and help decreased inflammation in our body.

So looking at these facts, are you reducing red-meat and butter, but replacing those tasty items with factory-made butter and rice-cakes? Cholesterol problems stem from eating too much fake fried food.

Myth No. 3: Cholesterol is the cause of heart disease

"The majority of the risk for heart disease is not explained by cholesterol," says Jeffrey Anderson, MD, a cardiologist and professor of medicine at the University of Utah. The problem is that not all doctors are caught up to speed with recent science. "What we've learned in recent years is that the problem is not just passive infiltration of cholesterol, but the fact that it provokes an inflammatory/immune process," Anderson explains. "Some people have a greater inflammatory process going on than others. We're still trying to track down the factors that make one group prone to this and others less so."

LDL is considered "bad" because small particles can creep into the lining of an artery and get deposited in its wall. The reason this happens is usually infection, inflammation or the occurrence of free radicals. The LDL that does get trapped in artery walls can get damaged then provoke an inflammatory response. These fats that are trapped are ingested by the immune system's white blood cells, which accumulate within the artery wall. Over the years, these areas of build-up form scab-like plaques; which partially or even completely block the artery; also known as atherosclerosis.

This leads to blockage or a ruptured build-up of plaque can cut off blood supply to the heart or brain, resulting in a heart attack or stroke.

The interesting part is that atherosclerosis is common in individuals with low LDL levels as well, perhaps because there is a unbalanced number of small LDL particles or because too many are being oxidized. Another interesting study finds that individuals with high LDL levels many times have perfectly healthy arteries. As with many diseases, genetics is one of the main culprits in causing heart disease.

Myth No. 4: Statin drugs are our friends

In July 2008, federal officials lowered the base for "desirable" low-density lipoprotein (LDL) levels, from 130mg per deciliter of blood to 100mg. The pharmaceutical companies loved hearing this because the change means that more patients will likely be urged to take statin drugs. But before reaching for that easy fix of prescription drugs, I want you to understand the issues that come along with them. Recent studies show that these statin drugs can lead to severe muscle damage. This problem is so serious Canadian regulators added special labels on Lipitor and other statin drugs.

Since, most people will still try to control their cholesterol with conventional low-fat dietary recommendations, pharmaceutical companies are raking in record profits selling statins, to an ever-increasing market, which now includes young children. Treating obese children with cholesterol drugs doesn't make any sense; the focus needs to be squarely on diet and exercise. I must emphasize, you couldn't live without LDL. The important piece is to find where that inflammation is coming from...could it be too much sugar???

Many critics of statins point to the lack of long-term safety data. Recent evidence suggests a host of potential statin side effects, such as muscle damage, dementia and impotence; and the possibility that artificially lowering children's cholesterol could delay normal growth and development; cholesterol is necessary for healthy cellular reproduction and hormone function.

Doctors and patients want a quick fix, so they use drugs to make the cholesterol score look better. The problem is that a better cholesterol score doesn't necessarily equate to better health. Statins are more like a band-aid. If you're doing things that are driving small particles that cause oxidation, like eating a high-sugar diet, you can take all the Lipitor medication you want and it won't work. We need to deal with the underlying cause. A study published in the January 2008 issue of the *American Heart Journal* found that nearly 75 percent of patients hospitalized for a heart attack had cholesterol levels that fell within the recommended guidelines. Plus, more than 20 percent of those studied were already taking statins. What is wrong with this picture?!

The take-home message is not to be afraid of your cholesterol. Instead, take a step back from low-fat diet fads and quick-fix drugs and look at the big picture. Make the lifestyle adjustments that are known to address the major underlying causes of heart disease; such as a high carbohydrate diets and lack of exercise.

WHERE DID THE MYTHS COME FROM?

In the late 1950's a researcher named Ancel Keys developed a theory called the lipid hypothesis stating that there is a direct relationship between the amount of saturated fat and cholesterol in the diet and the incidence of coronary heart. Numerous following studies have questioned his data. Even so, Keys' theory received far more publicity than those showing alternate facts. The food processing industries making fake butter and additives, the main beneficiaries of any research that found fault with competing traditional foods, began promoting and funding further research designed to support the lipid hypothesis. Sounds a bit fishy to me!

Nathan Pritikin is the name that nutritionists recognize as the man who started the "low-fat" craze. But Pritikin was a stronger advocated for elimination of sugar, white flour and all processed foods. He recommended fresh raw foods, whole grains and a strenuous exercise program; but it was the low-fat piece of his theory that received the most interest in the media. People following his ideas found that they lost weight and that their blood cholesterol levels declined. The reason this diet worked was likely due to many factors and having nothing to do with reduction in dietary fat. Pritikin was his first critic with the "fat-free" idea. Pritikin soon found that the fat-free diet had many problems, first was the fact that people just could not stay on it. People who were determined enough to remain fat-free for any length of time developed a lot of health problems including mineral deficiencies, low energy, difficulty in concentration, depression, and the side effect we all fear: weight gain.

Some "experts" guarantee us that the lipid hypothesis is backed by irrefutable scientific proof. In reality, there is very little proof to support the idea that a diet low in saturated fat and cholesterol reduces death from heart disease. Here are some surprising facts that the fake food manufactures would like to keep hidden… Let's look at 1920; heart disease was rare in America; so rare that when a young doctor named Paul Dudley White introduced the German electrocardiograph at Harvard University, he had a hard time finding subjects. The new machine showed the presence of arterial blockages, and providing early diagnosis of heart disease. White had to search for patients who could benefit from his new machine. During the next forty years, however, the incidence of coronary heart disease rose dramatically, so much that by the mid-fifties heart disease was the leading cause of death among Americans. Today heart disease causes at least 40% of all US deaths. So, if heart disease results from the consumption of saturated fats, you would expect to find an increase in animal fat in the American diet. **Actually, the reverse is true. From 1910 to 1970, the amount of animal fat in the American diet declined from 83% to 62%, and butter consumption dropped from 18 pounds per person per year to 4. During the same period the percentage of vegetable oils in the form of margarine, shortening and refined oils increased about 400% while the consumption of sugar and processed foods increased about 60%. WOW! I think we found the problem!**

STUDIES THAT CHALLENGE THE LIPID HYPOTHESIS

A Medical Research Council survey showed that men eating butter ran half the risk of developing heart disease as those using margarine. I wanted to "bold" that just to make sure you all caught that! I also love this fact… **Mother's milk provides a higher amount of cholesterol than almost any other food. It also contains over 50% of its calories as fat and most in the form of saturated fat. Both cholesterol and saturated fat are necessary for growth in babies and children, in particular the development of the brain. Yet, the American Heart Association is now advising a low-cholesterol, low-fat diet for children!** Commercial formulas are low in saturated fats and soy formulas are free of cholesterol. **A recent study connected low-fat diets with failure to thrive in children.** I think we can trust Mother Nature; she doesn't stand to profit from prescription drugs.

Numerous studies of patients with atherosclerosis, found no relationship between the level of cholesterol in the blood and the incidence of the artery disease. Additional surveys also didn't find a connection to blood cholesterol levels with "bad" dietary habits, such as use of red meat, animal fats, butter, eggs, whole milk, bacon, sausage and cheese.

If you have any question on saturated fats and heart disease here are some of my favorite studies to help clear up any confusion. A study comparing Jews when they lived in Yemen, their diets were filled with animal fats, to Yemenite Jews living in Israel, whose diets consisted of margarine and vegetable oils, revealed little heart disease or diabetes in the Jews living in Yemen, but high levels of both diseases in the Jews in Israel. The study also found that the Jews in Yemen consumed no sugar but those in Israel consumed sugar in amounts equaling 25-30% of total carbohydrate intake. Still not convinced? A study compared people in northern and southern India which showed a similar pattern. People in northern India eat 17 times more animal fat but have 7 times lower rate of heart disease than people in southern India.

Are you feeling better about eating that steak? If not, I have more...The Masai tribe of Africa survive largely on whole milk, blood and beef. They are free from coronary heart disease and have excellent blood cholesterol levels. Eskimos eat liberally of animal fats from fish and marine animals. On their native diet they are also free of disease. A study of the long-lived people of Soviet Georgia showed that those who eat the fattiest meat live the longest. In Okinawa, where the average life span for women is 84 years, the inhabitants eat generous amounts of pork and seafood and do all their cooking in lard. Mediterranean people have low rates of heart disease even though they eat a lot of saturated fat from lamb, sausage and goat cheese; up to 70% of their caloric intake. A study of Puerto Ricans found that, although they consume large amounts of animal fat, they have a very low incidence of colon and breast cancer.

So, I don't know about you, but I think I will keep enjoying my animal protein and steer clear of the sugar. I also like the studies including the French. If you have been lucky enough to travel to France, you have enjoyed the full-fat flavors of this country. The French diet is filled with saturated fats in the form of butter, eggs, cheese, cream, liver, meats and rich patés. Yet the French have a lower rate of coronary heart disease than many other western countries. This trend has recently gained international awareness as the French Paradox. Another thing to consider is that the French do suffer from many degenerative diseases, but they also eat large amounts of sugar and white flour and in recent years have increased their desire of processed "fake" foods. This is proven by the announcement of adding a McDonald's to the Louvre.

DANGERS OF VEGETABLE OILS

Americans have been given a lot of misinformation about the facts of saturated fats versus polyunsaturated oils. Some dietary "experts" tell us that the polyunsaturated oils are good for us and that the saturated fats cause heart disease. The result of this has been detrimental to our health; in the past we ate most of our fats in the saturated form, primarily from butter, lard, coconut oil and small amounts of olive oil. Since then, most of the fats in our diet are polyunsaturated vegetable oils from soy, corn, safflower and canola.

Excess use of polyunsaturated oils has been shown to increase a number of disease; including increased cancer, heart disease, immune system dysfunction, damage to the liver, reproductive organs and lungs, digestive disorders, decreased learning ability, impaired growth, and weight gain. Polyunsaturates cause so many health problems because they become oxidized or rancid when subjected to heat and oxygen when cooking. Rancid oils are free radicals, single atoms with an unpaired electron. These free-radicals are very chemically reactive. They attack cell membranes and cause damage in our DNA, causing alterations in tissue, blood vessels and skin. Free radical damage to the tissues and organs causes tumor growths, free radical damage to the skin causes wrinkles, and free radical damage in the blood vessels promotes the buildup of plaque. New evidence finds links to free radicals with autoimmune diseases such as arthritis and with Parkinson's disease, Alzheimer's, Lou Gehrig's disease and cataracts.

Problems linked with an excess of polyunsaturates are intensified by the fact that polyunsaturates in vegetable oils are in the form of unsaturated omega-6 fatty acid. Recent research has revealed that too much omega-6 in the diet creates an imbalance that can cause inflammation. This problem can result in increased tendency to form blood clots, high blood pressure, and irritation of the digestive tract, depressed immune function, sterility, cancer and weight gain.

The typical American diet is deficient in the unsaturated omega-3 linolenic acid. Omega 3s are vital for cell oxidation, metabolizing amino acids and decreasing inflammation. Omega 3 deficiencies have been associated with asthma, heart disease and learning deficiencies. All prepackaged foods are made with omega-6 vegetable oils. Another huge part of our imbalance of omega-3 to omega-6 is that current agricultural and manufacturing practices have reduced the amount of omega-3 fatty acids in commercially accessible vegetables, eggs, fish and meat. Organic eggs from hens allowed to feed on insects and green plants can contain omega-6 and omega-3 fatty acids in the beneficial ratio of approximately one-to-one; **but supermarket eggs come from corn-fed hens and can contain as much as 19 times more omega-6 than omega-3!**

BENEFITS OF SATURATED FATS

Saturated fats are not the cause of our modern diseases. On the contrary, they play a lot of vital roles in our body chemistry:

- Saturated fatty acids make up at least 50% of the cell membranes. They are what create our cells necessary stiffness and integrity.
- They play a vital role in the health of our bones. For calcium to be effectively incorporated into the skeletal structure, at least 50% of the dietary fats should be saturated.
- They guard the liver from alcohol and other toxins, such as **Tylenol**.
- They improve the immune system.
- Saturated fats have antimicrobial properties, which protect us against harmful microorganisms in the digestive tract.

BENEFITS OF CHOLESTEROL

Our blood vessels become damaged in a number of ways-through irritations caused by free radicals, or because they are structurally weak-and when this happens, the body's natural healing substance steps in to repair the damage; causing us to make more cholesterol. Cholesterol is manufactured in the liver and in our cells. Like saturated fats, the cholesterol we make and consume plays many vital roles:

- Cholesterol, along with saturated fats, give our cells required stiffness and stability. When the diet contains an excess of polyunsaturated fats (vegetable oils or omega-6), instead of saturated fats in the cell membrane, the cell walls become flabby. If this happens, cholesterol from the blood drives into the tissues to give them structural integrity. This is why serum cholesterol levels may go down temporarily when we replace saturated fats with polyunsaturated fats in the diet.

- Cholesterol is vital for production and function of serotonin receptors in the brain. Serotonin is the body's "feel-good" chemical. Low cholesterol levels have been linked to depression and aggression. Anti-depressants often don't work for patients that are on vegetarian diets.

- Mother's milk is particularly high in cholesterol and has an important enzyme that assists the baby in using this nutrient. Babies and children need foods high in cholesterol to guarantee proper development of the brain and nervous system.

- Cholesterol acts as a precursor to important hormones that help us deal with stress and protect the body against cancer and heart disease. It is also important to our sex hormones like androgen, testosterone, estrogen and progesterone.

- Cholesterol is necessary for us to use vitamin D; which is an essential fat-soluble vitamin needed for healthy bones and nervous system, insulin production, reproduction and immune system function, proper growth, mineral metabolism, and muscle tone.

- Bile is vital for digestion and assimilation of fats in the diet; which is made from cholesterol that we eat.

- Current studies are now showing that cholesterol performs as an antioxidant; which is why cholesterol levels go up with age. As an antioxidant, it protects us against free radical damage that leads to heart disease and cancer.

- Dietary cholesterol helps maintain the health of the intestinal wall. People on low-cholesterol vegetarian diets often develop leaky gut syndrome and other intestinal disorders.

Cholesterol can become damaged by exposure to heat and oxygen. This oxidized cholesterol tends to promote damage to the arterial cells and cause buildup of plaque in the arteries. Damaged cholesterol is found in powdered milk; which is added to reduced-fat milks to give them body. That is why I NEVER suggest drinking skim milk! It is also found in powdered eggs and in meats that have been heated to high temperatures in frying and other high-temperature processes. So fast food items come into play here.

Hypothyroidism can result in high cholesterol levels. When thyroid function is poor, usually due to a diet low in usable iodine, fat-soluble vitamins and high in sugar, the blood gets filled with cholesterol as a protective mechanism, providing a large amount of minerals needed to heal tissues. Hypothyroid individuals are particularly susceptible to infections, heart disease and cancer.

TRANS-FATS AND HOW THEY ARE MADE – YUCK!

Hydrogenation is the process that turns polyunsaturates, normally liquid at room temperature, into fats that are solid at room temperature; enter "I Can't Believe It's Not Butter"…I can! To produce them, food producers begin with the cheapest oils-soy, corn, cottonseed or canola, already rancid and full of free-radicals. Then they mix it with tiny **metal particles-usually nickel oxide.** The oil with its metal is then put into hydrogen gas in a high-temperature machine. Next, soap-like products and starch are added into the mixture to give it a better consistency; the oil is yet again subjected to high temperatures when it is cleaned by steaming. **This removes its unpleasant odor. Margarine's natural color, an unappetizing grey, is removed by bleach.** Dyes and strong flavors are then be added to make it look like butter. The finished product is then squashed and packaged in blocks or tubs and sold as a "cholesterol-lowering" health food. Yikes! I'm sticking with yummy butter.

Partially hydrogenated margarines are worse for you than the extremely refined vegetable oils which they come from because of chemical processes that occur during the hydrogenation process. The extremely high temperatures, and the nickel that causes the hydrogen atoms to change position makes these items extremely harmful to our heart, cells and waist line! Before hydrogenation, pairs of hydrogen atoms occur together on the chain; this pattern is commonly found in nature. After hydrogenation, one hydrogen atom of the pair is moved to the other side so that the molecule straightens. This is called the *trans* formation, and rarely found in nature. These factory-made *trans* fats are toxins to the body, but sadly our digestive system does not identify them as such. Instead of being eliminated, *trans* fats are included into cells as if they were natural fats and **our cells become partially hydrogenated!** Once our cells become hydrogenated, our metabolism is slowed, not to mention the scary connection to cancer and other diseases.

In the 1940's, studies found a powerful connection between trans-fats and cancer. Until lately saturated fats were usually lumped together with trans-fats in U.S. data bases that scientists use to connect dietary trends with diseases. And this is where a lot of misinformation comes in about natural saturated fats.

Altered partially hydrogenated fats actually block use of essential fatty acids, causing many harmful effects including cancer, atherosclerosis, diabetes, obesity, immune system dysfunction, birth defects, decreased visual acuity, sterility, low-birth-weight babies, and hardships with lactation. Yet, look at the false advertising, hydrogenated fats promote themselves as health foods. The attractiveness of partially hydrogenated margarine over butter represents a victory of advertising fraudulence over common sense. Your best defense is to eat things as close to nature as possible; the less the ingredients, the better.

BUTTER VS. MARGARINE

Claims that butter causes chronic high cholesterol have not been proven by research; actually studies have shown that stearic acid, found in beef fat, lowers cholesterol. Even though the food manufacturers are catching on…so are the advertising laws…they can advertise "NO TRANS-FATS," but the law states they can lower the serving size as tiny as they want and as long as there is less than one gram per serving. The new soft margarines, while lower in hydrogenated fats, are still produced from harmful vegetable oils and include many additives to make that junk taste better.

Nutrients in Butter

The powerful food advertisers have been very effective claiming that butter is hazardous, when in fact it is a valued part of many established diets and includes important nutrients. Here is a list of some:

Fat-Soluble Vitamins: These include vitamin A, D, K and E along with their naturally occurring cofactors needed to gain the greatest effect. Butter is our best source of these important nutrients. Go figure, butter has the best source of vitamin A, most readily absorbed and utilized, than from any other source. Fortunately, these fat-soluble vitamins are quite stable and survive the pasteurization process.

An important researcher named, Dr. Weston Price, studied remote traditional people around the world. He found that butter was a staple in many native diets and he did not find any who consumed polyunsaturated oils. One important piece to note it that the butter was deep yellow and made from grass-fed cows, not corn-fed beef, like the butter from our main supermarkets. When Dr. Price studied the grass-fed butter he found that it was very high in all fat-soluble vitamins, particularly vitamin A. According to Dr. Price, without them, we are not able to use the other minerals we eat, no matter how plentiful they may be in our diets. He also believed the fat-soluble vitamins are necessary for absorption of water-soluble vitamins. Vitamins A and D are essential for growth, for healthy bones, for proper development of the brain and nervous systems. It is also important for reproduction; it brings out male and female sexual characteristics. These essential nutrients are especially beneficial for children and expectant mothers. As the use of butter in America has declined, sterility rates and problems with sexual development have increased. **When animals consume butter substitutes, their growth is stunted and they are unable to sustain reproduction.**

Not all the societies Dr. Price studied ate butter; but they went to great lengths to obtain foods high in fat-soluble vitamins; such as, fish, shellfish, organ meats, blubber of sea animals and insects. These isolated societies recognized the importance of these items in the diet and liberally ate the animal products containing them. Dr. Price found that their diet provided about ten times more fat soluble vitamins than the American diet of the 1930's. This ratio is more extreme today since Americans have considerably reduced animal fat consumption.

Conjugated Linoleic Acid: Butter from pasture-fed cows also contains a form of linoleic acid called CLA; it helps build muscle and prevents weight gain. CLA also has strong cancer fighting properties. CLA disappears when cows are fed dry hay or processed feed; so spending a few extra dollars on grass-fed butter is worth it. It also tastes way better!

Lecithin: Lecithin is a large element of butter that helps in the absorption and digestion of cholesterol. This nutrient is also abundant in organic egg yolks.

Glycosphingolipids: This fat may be new to most of you. It is very helpful in preventing gastrointestinal infections, particularly in children and the elderly. For this reason, young **children who drink skimmed milk have diarrhea at rates up to five times greater than children who drink whole milk.**

Trace Minerals: Manganese, zinc, chromium and iodine are all helpful components of butter. In areas that didn't receive foods from the sea, iodine in butter protected against goiter. Butter is very rich in selenium, a trace mineral with antioxidant properties, having more per gram than herring or wheat germ.

CONQUERING HIGH CHOLESTEROL

Here are six ways to right-size your cholesterol, reduce your heart-disease risk factors and get a whole lot healthier in the process:

1. **Eat less sugar and flour.** Starch and sugars not only spark inflammation, they elevate triglycerides. Too many triglycerides in the blood impede the circulation of healthy cholesterol, causing the entire system to break down. When choosing grain products look for those made with whole and sprouted grains. Avoid cereals, cookies, cakes and other sweets, and minimize your intake of pastas and breads.

2. **Eat more non-starchy vegetables.** The antioxidants and phytonutrients in vegetables help protect cholesterol in the blood from free-radical damage. They are also high in fiber, which assists the body in ridding itself of cholesterol-laden bile. A Harvard Nurses' Health Study showed that participants who ate five or more servings of vegetables a day had a 25 percent lower risk of heart attack and stroke than those who ate the fewest servings.

3. **Eat quality fats and cut out trans-fats.** That means cutting trans-fats entirely, and avoiding high-fat processed and fried foods in favor of healthy, nutrient-dense whole foods. Enjoy nuts, seeds, fish, avocados and olive oil, and don't feel you need to cut out saturated fats entirely either. The body craves these and requires them for proper cell, nerve and brain function. Plus, when people don't satisfy their flavor and satisfaction desires for saturated fats, they'll often consume processed carbohydrates instead, thereby increasing insulin, weight gain and inflammation. When selecting meat and dairy choose minimally processed foods ideally from pastured, free-range and grass-fed animals. These have more nutrients the body needs and fewer pro-inflammatory fats. Eating eggs are fine too, even the yolks! **Research published in the AMERICAN JOURNAL OF CLINICAL NUTRITION shows that people eating up to seven eggs a week are no more likely to experience heart attacks or strokes than those who eat less than an egg a week.**

4. **Get more fiber.** Eating more soluble fiber is one of the easiest ways to naturally lower your cholesterol. Fiber binds to bile, which is composed of cholesterol and triglycerides, and escorts it (along with other inflammatory toxins), out of the body. The liver then produces fresh bile, making use of cholesterol and triglycerides that would otherwise accumulate in the bloodstream. By eating two high-fiber foods a day can make a big difference. Nuts, flaxseeds, vegetables and coconut flour are all high in fiber. Flaxseeds are extra special because they have hormone-regulating properties that help regulate insulin and make sure cholesterol stays in check. Not a big fan of flaxseeds? Another option is to add 2 teaspoons of psyllium husks to your diet.

5. **Exercise.** Moderate to intense exercise lowers cholesterol overall and raises the relative levels of protective HDL. Exercise also helps reduce excess inflammatory effects of stress and help reduce weight. A 2006 Duke study that examined the effects of exercise on inactive, overweight adults found that, after six months, many of the factors putting them at risk for heart disease had reversed.

6. **Consider CoQ10:** CoEnzymeQ10 is a powerful vitamin-like nutrient that helps increase the mitochondria in our cells. The mitochondrion is

the part of the cell that burns fat and lowers triglycerides. Add 400mg at breakfast.

To sum up all the confusion about saturated fats and cholesterol, I want you to leave this chapter realizing that our choice of fats and oils is of extreme importance to our wellbeing. Infants and small children, benefit from *more* fat in the diet rather than less. Being aware of the types of fats we consume must be of utmost importance. Avoid all processed foods containing harmful hydrogenated fats and polyunsaturated oils; instead of buying pre-packaged cookies, make you own with real butter! They taste better anyway. Use oils like extra virgin olive oil and small amounts of unrefined flax seed oil. Start experimenting with coconut oil for your pie crusts and baked goods. Use animal fats for occasional frying. Don't be afraid of egg yolks and other animal fats that will keep our bodies strong and beautiful. Lastly, use good organic butter, with the assurance that it is a wholesome, omega 3-filled safe food for you and your family.

The best way to treat heart disease is to enjoy a diet that provides animal foods that provide vitamins B_6 and B_{12}; bolster thyroid function by daily use of iodized sea salt; and to avoid vitamin and mineral deficiencies, specifically magnesium and vitamin E and C, that make the artery walls vulnerable to ruptures and the buildup of plaque. More importantly we need to eliminate processed foods containing refined carbohydrates, oxidized cholesterol (skim milk) and free-radical-containing vegetable oils that cause inflammation in the body.

CHAPTER 5

EXERCISE AND ENERGY

I get a lot of questions on how much fat is in my recipes. Why don't I label it? Well, because fat is my source of energy. I even run marathons with this diet and I never 'hit the wall.'

People often complain of low energy when they first start a low carb diet because they are "sugar-burners." This is not only inefficient, but very detrimental to our health. For one reason, cancer LOVES sugar! This is why cancer patients drink a huge glass of glucose to see where the caner is in their body. Cancer feeds on sugar, if you eat more sugar, the more the cancer grows.

Energy actually comes from a chemical we produce in our body called adenosine triphosphate (ATP). We can produce energy 2 ways: anaerobic and aerobic.

1. Anaerobic ('without oxygen') bacteria break down glucose to produce energy. Our cells can use this method.
2. Aerobic ('with oxygen'). All human and animal life requires oxygen to function.

As we breathe in oxygen, we carry it through the hemoglobin to the mitochondria (the powerhouse of our cells) where we burn fat and produce energy. The more mitochondria you have, the more energy and therefore, more fat burning. AND the more healthy fats = more mitochondria. You can also increase the amount of mitochondria with certain supplements which I discuss in the Supplement Chapter.

*Please note that if you have a food allergy, you can't absorb iron properly which will inhibit you from carrying oxygen to the mitochondria. This will cause exhaustion due to low ATP production along with other problems.

Energy Can Come From:
1. Glucose: created with carbohydrates and protein
2. Fats, both from the diet and from stored body fats
3. Ketones which are derived from the metabolism of fats

GLUCOSE and ENERGY = EAT PROTEIN

Some cells, such as the kidneys have very little mitochondria so they don't use fat for energy, so this is why eating protein for glucose is important. If we go too long without eating, we maintain glucose levels by breaking down glycogen in muscle proteins with a process called gluconeogenesis. BUT this is not healthy. There is a detrimental phenomenon called SARCOPENIA where we lose 1% of our muscle every year starting at age 25, which is terrible because 1 pound of muscle burns 50 calories and 1 pound of fat burns only 2...even when we sleep!

So we don't want to be cannibals to our muscles. Eating adequate amounts of protein will produce glucose (healthy carbs such as non-starchy veggies and almond/coconut flour will too). Our cells need a steady supply of protein to sustain a healthy structure. Any protein over and above 1 to 1.5 grams/kilogram of lean body weight/day can be used as a source of glucose. Anything less will cause you to start eating healthy muscle tissue. When you eat protein, you convert about 58% to glucose. So 100g of protein will produce 58 grams of glucose.

KETONES and ENERGY = EAT HEALTHY FATS

So if you want to stop being a "sugar burner" you must derive energy from another source. Enter fat. When we start eating a healthy low carb diet, our bodies slowly switch from burning sugar to burning fat. This is where eating becomes an "art." Energy must be derived from healthy fatty acids and ketones produced from foods such as coconut oil. At first the body will feel lethargic due to the mechanisms switching over; burning sugar is easy, burning fat takes a few days to adapt.

The brain prefers to use ketones instead of glucose for energy (in Alzheimer's the brain can no longer convert glucose for energy, coconut oil is VERY healthy for these patients!).

Eating a very low carbohydrate diet stimulates the production of ketones from body fat; which is why people lose so much weight on this diet. Cutting out carbs and increasing protein also leads to a lower insulin level in the blood. A normal blood sugar is 1 TEASPOON of sugar in your blood. Many Americans consume over 63 teaspoons a day! If you can conquer a normal blood sugar, it reduces the problems associated with high insulin levels; insulin resistance, leptin resistance, high blood pressure, Metabolic Syndrome, weight gain, sleep issues...

To produce ketones, focus on carbs being only 10% of your total intake. For diabetics, the level may need to be lower to counteract insulin resistance. Typical levels of carb intake for a type-2 diabetic are around 50 grams per day; the level should be lower still at about 30 grams a day for a type-1 diabetic. Here is a good ratio to follow for calories/macro-nutrient consumption:

10-15% carbs
20-39% protein
60-70% fat

Extra Fat Bur⌐

If you have rea⌐ by Suzanne Som⌐ read about the m⌐ the human growth hormone that she injects into her body every day. The human growth hormone mobilizes fat (burns fat) to raise blood glucose when low. Sounds great, but you don't need to inject this hormone to enhance your levels. Naturally growth hormone is released during long-wave sleep in the first few hours after you go to bed at night. So you burn fat at night! BUT if blood glucose is high, growth hormone release is inhibited almost completely; which results in zero fat burn at night. This means that you shouldn't eat for about 2-3 hours before you go to sleep to maximize the HGH production and fat burn. You can also increase your human growth hormone when you lift heavy weights…so increase those weights!

So, please listen: don't eat just lean proteins! It is not tolerated well in our body. It leads to nausea in as little as

..e days. A high healthy fat diet, however, is the traditional diet to sustain for a lifetime. Eating only lean protein causes excess intake of nitrogen, which leads to hyperammonaemia, which is a buildup of ammonia in the bloodstream and is toxic to the brain. Many traditional societies survived on a purely animal product diet, which was naturally high in fat...they didn't have George Foreman Grills.

Our paleo ancestors actually consumed more fat than protein; with a ratio of about 80% calories from fat and 20% from protein. During prolonged periods of starvation or something such as marathon running, fatty acids are converted into ketones, the preferred energy source for highly active tissues like those found in the heart and muscles. Ketones provide a long lasting energy to all cells with mitochondria. Ketones are used to generate ATP. If you use glucose for energy, it needs the intervention of bacteria, ketones can be used directly.

*Note: Using a quality REAL salt is also essential for electrolyte balance. We start skipping the salt and we get low energy. I'm not talking about pre-packaged and fast food junk salt. A Celtic Sea Salt filled with minerals will help with energy.

What exercise does for metabolism

I know that there will be individuals reading this, telling themselves that they don't have time to exercise, or don't really feel they need to, but this part of the brain is sabotaging their efforts to improve their health. This is the same part of the brain that tells you that your healthy eating plan can wait until Monday, or that one more cookie won't make any difference. We all have coping strategies to rationalize choices we make, even though we know that what we are saying to ourselves are just excuses. The trick is to learn to realize when you are lying to yourself and not listen to the voice of negativity. This is very important in the process to make positive changes in any area of your life including exercise. I love this quote: **"Movement is medicine for changing a person's physical, emotional, and mental state."**

Recent studies found that exercise is more helpful in treating depression than antidepressant medications. Beyond that, we all know that exercise helps us lose weight and build lean muscle. Hmmm... exercise helps reshape the body, brighten the spirits, and sharpen the mind. I'm sold!

I feel there are 3 very important types of exercise to include in your own workout plan. These don't need to be performed every day, nor should they. You must consider your cardiovascular exercise to elevating your heart rate, muscular exercise to strengthen your muscles, and yoga exercises to improve your posture, balance, and range of motion around your joints and decrease risk of injury. Each area is very important and should be included in your exercise routine.

Strength Training

I originally started this chapter with cardiovascular exercise, but I realized that starting with the most important version of exercise would be more fitting. Most women are using their valuable time with cardiovascular or aerobic exercise and I was one of them. I would run for 12 miles a day, run races that were 26.2 miles long, but the scale didn't budge. I finally started a fitness class called BodyPump and the weight started to melt off. I stopped running so much and replaced it with weight training.

Still scared to change? Check this out:

Studies compared dieters who lifted 3 times a week with those who did aerobics.

- Both groups consumed the same number of calories
- Both lost the same amount of weight
    BUT...
- Weight lifters lost all Fat
- Aerobics lost a lot of valuable muscle
- Also found weight lifters lost intra-abdominal fat easier
- Fat associated with diseases (diabetes to cancer)

MUSCLE IS also DENSER than fat. So even though the groups lost the same amount of weight...the weight lifters jeans fit better!

Women often shy away from strength training for a variety of reasons. There are a lot of myths floating around. Here are some of the top myths that I want to clear up:

Myth 1: For weight loss, I should only do cardio exercise.

While cardio exercise is important for losing weight, it isn't the only type of exercise that can help you lose fat. Strength training helps you preserve the muscle you have as well as increase your muscle mass and the more muscle you have, the more calories you'll burn all day long. Muscle is more active than fat.

In fact, a pound of muscle can burn around 50 calories a day while a pound of fat burns only 2 calories a day. Muscle is denser than fat and takes up less space. That means when you lose fat and gain muscle, you'll be slimmer and trimmer. Plenty of people, especially women, avoid strength training like the plague, either because they think they'll gain weight or because they like cardio better. But strength training has a number of benefits such as:

- It builds lean muscle tissue
- It strengthens muscles, bones and connective tissue
- It keeps your body strong and injury-free for your cardio workouts
- It raises metabolism

Myth 2: To "tone" my muscles, I should use lighter weights and high reps.

This is another myth that I refer to as, 'The Pink Dumbbell Myth' that is often told by magazines and infomercials, convincing us that we should use lighter weights (pink dumbbells) for higher reps to tone our bodies. There's also a belief that this approach somehow burns more fat and that women should lift weights this way to avoid getting big and bulky.

The truth is that this type of strength training doesn't burn more fat and the only way it will 'tone' your body is if you've created a calorie deficit that allows you to lose body fat. Using lighter weights for higher reps will help you increase muscular endurance and it does have a place in training routines, but that lean, defined look comes from losing body fat, which means heavy weights = more fat burning!

- ✓ For strength gains: 1-6 reps, heavy weight
- ✓ For gaining muscle: 8-12 reps, medium-heavy weights
- ✓ For endurance: 12-16 reps (or more), medium weights

No matter what range you choose, you should always lift enough weight that you can ONLY complete the desired reps. If you're doing 12 bicep curls, choose a weight that allows you to 12 reps with good form. If you can do more than that, increase your weight. You need to have your muscles burn at the end to increase Human Growth Hormone production, which increases our fat burning. Body builders get their physique by lifting weights for about 4 hours a day and eating totally "clean." Lifting heavy weights for 45 minutes 3 times a week isn't going to create that look.

Myth 3: Strength training makes women bulk up

This is another popular myth that continues regardless of the fact that women don't have the amount of testosterone required to build huge muscles. In fact, even men struggle to gain muscle which is one reason steroids are so popular with men who want to build big muscles.

Lifting heavy weights can benefit both men and women and, in fact, challenging your body with heavy weights is the only way you'll really see results and get stronger. I've been lifting heavy weights for years and have never even come close to looking like a bodybuilder; most women who lift weights would agree. Remember, muscle takes up less space than fat. When you add muscle, that helps you lose fat (along with your cardio

Wear a Pedometer:
We have an odometer in the car recording the miles our cars have traveled. Similarly, pedometers measure our steps. Walking 10,000 steps a day will help you burn about 300 to 400 calories. Walking is a physical activity and every activity will burn calories. A pedometer can enhance your motivation to increase your step quota every day. Focus on just one day at a time. Over time, you will find yourself going for an extra walk, taking extra steps from the parking lot and expending just a few more calories here and there. These small changes add up over the course of the year leading to stable, lifelong results.

Metabolism and Low Calorie Diets

Research has demonstrated that one of the most important benefits of resistance exercise in a weight loss program is the conservation of muscle mass, even on very low-calorie diets. In addition, scientist Andrew Hill has found that diet only programs can lower a person's resting metabolic rate by 20%; which is approximately 300 fewer calories expended per day! Research shows that strength training is the best protective intervention to maintain metabolism during a caloric restrictive diets. When we go on calorie restricted diets, most people lose valuable muscle, but adding strength training helps to keep that muscle and burn fat instead!

and healthy diet, of course), which means you'll be leaner and more defined.

Are you gaining weight with strength training? One reason women say their pants fit tighter after lifting heavier weights is that **they are over consuming carbohydrates. Carbs will increase insulin which will cause muscle to grow (good) BUT it will hinder fat-loss (bad). Don't grab oatmeal and skim milk after all your hard work, use a protein source to re-fuel your muscles and keep the insulin from rising too much. Marathoners are often guilty of this...did you know a pound of fat is 3,500 calories and if you run a full marathon you only burn about 2,500 calories? That's not even one pound.** You need a lot of energy to finish a marathon, which is why I used to gain weight pushing myself through races. Learning the proper ways to fuel your body is essential for your health and outward appearance. It takes 3,500 calories to burn one pound of fat...that is A LOT. So don't think that since you performed a 'kick-butt' workout you can have a bag of Twizzlers.

I know those of you who are Gary Taube's fans will think I am wrong, but I have seen the benefits of exercise and cardio. Cardiovascular exercise is necessary for a number of reasons: First, it improves the efficiency of your heart and lungs and enables your body to intake and use greater amounts of oxygen. If your body is able to pump more oxygen you will be less likely to get out of breath so fast. You will be able to sustain physical activity for longer durations and your heart and lungs will be stronger. This is known as cardiovascular fitness; Lance Armstrong is a freak of nature because his oxygen consumption is so high.

EXERCISE MAKES YOU A BETTER 'FAT BURNER'

Studies signify that a number of metabolic changes occur with cardiovascular exercise that uniquely enhance fat metabolism, including the following:

1. A major boost in the number and size of the mitochondria. The mitochondrion is the only place in a cell where fat is burned and oxidized. It is the cell's 'fat burning furnace.'
2. An increase in the oxidative enzymes that 'speed up' the transport of fatty acids molecules

When you exercise at a high intensity, changes begin to happen in your body. Your body creates more mitochondria in the muscles and the mitochondria are responsible for processing oxygen. To cut a long story short, your body will only use fat in the presence of oxygen, so the higher your body's ability to process oxygen, the greater your capability to burn fat! **Please be advised that when your body consumes more oxygen you also create more free radicals within your body. Free radicals are unstable particles, which damage healthy cells in a process called oxidation or free-radical damage. It is universally believed that we need to ensure that athletes take in higher quantities of antioxidants to remove free radicals and defend our bodies from degenerative diseases. (See Supplements Chapter)** to be used for energy during cardiovascular exercise.

3. An increased oxygen delivery through blood flow which helps the cell oxidize and burn fat more proficiently.

4. An amplified sensitivity of muscles and fat cells to epinephrine helps increase the release of triglycerides into the blood and the muscle to clear them from our body.

5. Specialized protein transporters also move fatty acids into the muscle cell at a higher rate, making fat more available for energy.

6. A boost in the amount of fatty acids allowed into the muscle, which also makes fat more available for energy.

I love this information; it shows that with consistent, progressive cardiovascular exercise we can truly expand our body's to be awesome 'fat burners'. It is very gratifying to know that when our bodies are tired and we want to stop exercising, we are creating more 'fat burning' furnaces (mitochondria) in our bodies to push us through the pain!

FAT BURNING ZONE

Some people believe in order to maximize your fat burning you need to find your "fat burning zone." The fat burning zone is the zone at which you are doing enough work to burn fat. Your heart rate determines which zone you are in. There has been some controversy whether or not this is true...but it may be worth trying. To find your fat burning zone it takes a little math. The fat burning zone formula is the following:

Fat burning zone=220-(Your Age) x (.75)

The number you get will give you an approximate rate of how fast your heart should be beating per minute. For example, a 20-year-old would need to reach a pulse in the neighborhood of 150 beats per minute in order to be in the fat burning zone. This is not an absolute figure, this is an estimate. Trying to have your pulse plus or minus 10 beats from the number you receive from the formula provides that you will be burning fat. One problem I find with this is that you will also need a heart rate monitor to determine if you are in that zone while exercising. I also think that there are more efficient ways to burn more calories.

INTERVAL TRAINING

I think it is important to note that we should focus workout plans on burning the most calories possible whether it is harder, longer or a combination of both. To burn more fat, burn more calories and that is why the "fat burning zone" isn't always the best. My favorite way to burn "free" calories is known as Interval Training. Not only do you burn a lot more calories while you're performing interval training, you also stimulate your metabolism to a far greater degree than with lower intensity training, which is traditionally known for fat loss.

Your body will burn more calories after exercise when you use intervals than it does after you do slow consistent cardio and your metabolism will stay high. This is referred to this as the "after-burn" effect. How do you do intervals? Well, you could sprint for 30 seconds and walk for 90 seconds and repeat that for 6 sets. Within that short time frame the intervals will cause your muscles to go crazy with activity; I call it a metabolic disturbance. This crazy metabolism boost causes lots of calorie burning after exercise to get your body back to normal. The result is you would end up burning more fat and more calories in the post-exercise period as your body tries to get things under control.

The exercise after-burn is the number of calories expended above resting values after a workout. Although intensity dependent, both aerobic and resistance training programs may elicit 150-250 (primarily fat) calories post workout. One pound of fat is equal to 3,500 calories. If you exercise 5 days/week, over the course of the year the "after burn" would be calculated as follows: 5 workouts/week x 52 weeks x 100 EPOC calories/ workout total 26,000 calories or 7 lbs of fat ("afterburn" minimum is 100 calories, work harder and reach 250 calories...awesome) that's meaningful!

You can wipe out an entire workout's benefits in less than a minute simply by eating garbage. Without some structure and discipline to your nutrition, there is nothing that even my programs can do to help you lose fat. So include nutrition and interval training. These are the two anti-calorie counting methods that will help you lose fat and get lean. Good nutrient timing strategies are based on the fact that the body best handles different types of food at different times of the day. One of the most important nutrient timing strategies dictates that you should eat most of your non-fruit and veggie carbohydrates immediately after exercise. This rule is especially important for people trying to lose weight. If you haven't just exercised, put down the pasta, the breads, the rice, and step away from the table.

WHY HIGH-INTENSITY INTERVAL TRAINING IS AWESOME:

1. It saves time. If you normally spend an hour and a half in the gym following the "fat burning zone" philosophy, you'll work yourself just as hard in 45 minutes with interval training.

2. Higher intensities stimulate your metabolism far more AFTER the workouts than lower intensity training. This means you continue to burn calories and fat for long periods after you're done training. Not so with the "fat burning zone." This is called the 'afterburn,' which can burn an extra 150-250 calories after you stop exercising.

3. It combats boredom. It's fun, and the time flies by during each session, because you're working in cycles of high and low intensity work instead of spending a long period of time at any one activity. I like to make a playlist of songs to match my intensity of the workout; a warm-up song, a fast paced song, followed by a recovery paced song, and repeat!

Interval training is based on a very simple concept: go fast then go slow. Repeat. It sounds simple, but this formula has an incredible number of potential variations and strategies. To begin, start your workout at an easy pace and slowly increase your heart rate for at least five minutes. You can monitor this by using a heart rate monitor or just use a "rate of perceived exertion" test: judging how hard your workout is by a rate of 1-10 (1 is resting, 10 is hardest possible). When you're warmed up, you're ready for an explosion of high intensity work. Break into a jog or a sprint, depending on what "high intensity" means to you; your "rate of perceived exertion" should be around 8 and you shouldn't be able to carry on a conversation.

During the high intensity periods, you're diminishing your body's ability to swap oxygen and carbon dioxide. You begin to feel the "burn" as your body eliminates lactic acid and your muscles start to lose their ability to contract. You are working so hard, you aren't physically able to continue this level of intensity for long. After a few minutes, reduce the intensity level to something that you could maintain for a longer period, but don't slow down too much that your pulse dips too low because you will lose the aerobic effect completely. This period is called the "active recovery period". Your body increases the exchange of oxygen and carbon dioxide to deliver nutrients to your muscles. The 'lactic acid' burn diminishes and your breathing rate slows down a bit. After you complete this period for a few minutes, you have accomplished one cycle.

Repeat this process of feeling the burn and recovering for at least thirty minutes. The high intensity periods should be shorter than the active recovery periods, particularly when you first start. For example when you begin to introduce your body to interval training; walk for five minutes, then run for one. As you become more proficient, increase the time you spend in high intensity periods.

Interval training helps us lose weight faster in many ways. Interval training challenges your aerobic and anaerobic systems at the same time; therefore, you're improving your body's capacity to burn calories at a higher rate. You're also adding new muscle, which speeds up your metabolism of fat even at rest. You're getting an aerobic workout that burns lots of calories. Interval training is also effective at pushing beyond plateaus in weight loss. Your body becomes a valuable fat-burning machine.

Many scientists have proven this theory. One study followed a group of overweight women and assigned them to one of two groups. The first group worked out using high intensity intervals, which involved 2 minutes of maximum effort followed by 3 minutes at a lower intensity. Group two worked out at a constant pace for the whole time. The lengths of the workouts were varied so that both groups burned 300 calories. The outcome found that fitness levels in the interval group improved by 13%. No improvements were found in the steady state group. The first group also continued to burn extra calories after the workout was finished; known as the "afterburn." Remember the "afterburn" can help us burn an extra 150-250 calories after our workout while at rest! When you push your muscles to the point of exhaustion it takes a lot of effort to repair them.

I also want to point out a few tips that can increase fat burning. Aerobic exercise should be performed at the certain times to maximize your efforts; granted these tips will not work for everyone since we need to fit in our exercise when we can and some people may want to enhance their performance rather than burn fat. These are "fat burning" tips, not "performance enhancing" tips. If you are looking to train for a race, you will want to train with food to increase your speed. But if "fat loss" is your goal…check this out!

1. **In The Morning On An Empty Stomach**: The best time to burn fat is to perform aerobic exercise is first thing in the morning on an empty stomach after drinking a large glass of water, or a little coffee too, in order to avoid dehydration. You burn 300% more body fat in the morning on an empty stomach than at any other time in the day because your body does not have any glycogen or stored carbohydrates/sugar in the liver to burn. When this happens, your body has to go directly into the fat stores in order to get the energy necessary to complete the activity. You also increase your human growth hormone levels; which is the fat-burning hormone. The human growth hormone and insulin counteract each other. If one is high, the other is low…like a see-saw. So if you eat something, especially carbohydrates before a workout you will be spiking your insulin levels, meaning your growth hormone levels will be low. If you are diabetic or have other medical issues, this is not a healthy practice. This suggestion is only for people who have no medical conditions and are not training to win any races.

2. **Right after Weight Training**: After lifting weights is another great time to maximize your fat burning efforts. If you can't do cardiovascular exercise in the morning it takes your body around 20 to 30 minutes to start burning fat because that it how long it takes the body to exhaust its glycogen stores and switch to start burning fat instead. Performing weight training first helps do deplete your glycogen stores faster. Lifting weights first also gives you lots of energy to focus on correct posture to decrease the chance of injury.

3. **Change the Exercise:** Changing up aerobic exercises is essential because our muscles get use to repetitions; workouts get easier and our muscles don't have to work as hard…they know what to expect; therefore, you burn less calories. Changing activities makes your muscles and brain work harder and this causes an increase in heart rate, which means an increase in calories burned.

4. **Change the Amount of Time during Exercise:** This is important because we want to prevent our body from adjusting to a constant length of the activity. Just as in the type of exercise, as soon as the body adapts, it is easier for our muscles to perform. This is good for our performance, but it will be tougher to reach the fat burning zone and therefore changing the duration is important. Sometimes I like to split my workout in two; a shorter fat burning interval in the morning, then another short burst before dinner. Take that "thunder thighs,"…that was my childhood nickname!

Cardio can help us all maximize our metabolism in many ways. Just make sure you push your body outside of its usual relaxed state and overload your muscles; feel the burn! Overloading a muscle encourages it to work harder than it normally would and this also applies to your heart muscle. With all the benefits of exercise, I am hooked for life. It lifts my spirits on a bad day, it lets me enjoy a bowl of ice cream once in a while, it is fun to socialize with friends…the list goes on.

It is also important to remember that one pound of fat is 3, 500 calories. This is A LOT! Just because we go for a 30 minute run, doesn't mean we are allowed dessert every day. If you want to drop weight, that run burned only about 300 calories…we need to get another 3,200 calorie deficit to lose 1 pound. Don't be discouraged, just stay the course. Reward yourself in other ways; I suggest my clients to plan a massage that lasts an hour and look forward to that as a way to reward your muscles for all their hard work instead of a calorie busting brownie that lasts for 5 minutes.

Circuit Training: Strength and Cardio!

Circuit training revs up your metabolism and extends your endurance. It is a combination of strength and cardiovascular training. If you're looking for a workout that provides all-over fitness benefits, look no further than circuit training. A circuit workout is a resistance workout with little to no rest between exercises. The absence of long rest periods makes circuit training as effective as a cardio-based high-intensity interval workout (HIIT); which raises your heart rate like a cardio workout and boosts metabolism by building muscles. HIIT burns a ton of calories, and not just during the workout, but for hours afterward…the "afterburn" effect. Circuit training combines the benefits of cardio exercise and resistance exercise better than any other activity.

Choosing multi-joint movements that use a lot of different muscles in one activity is the most beneficial. Your metabolism and heart rate are directly related to the total volume of muscle mass you stimulate. So, choosing multi-joint, whole-body movements burns more calories and stimulates your brain and muscles to think harder, improving movement skills. Minimizing rest time between exercises is as important as the exercises themselves. The more downtime you have between movements, the more your heart rate and metabolic rate decrease. You can choose to do strength-focused circuits, cardio-focused circuits or a combination of both.

I love a class at my local YMCA called, "Bootcamp." My instructor is an Olympic Gold medalist from the USA women's hockey team. She is very inspirational. She designs her class to be different every day, but it is based off of a circuit training workout. In our group of 30 die-hard Bootcamp fans, she has us rotate stations that include one strength training activity and one cardiovascular activity. One example of a station is; bicep curls for one person and explosive step-ups over en elevated step for person two (switching every minute, two minutes or whatever she has planned for the day). Once you are done with that station, we quickly do 15 push-ups, sit-ups or squats, and then move onto the next heart pumping station.

Here is an efficient way to burn that fat:

Warm-Up for 5 minutes, then Jog for 5minutes

✓ Do 10 push-ups, then 10 sit ups
✓ 9 push-ups, 9 sit ups
✓ 8 push-ups, 8 sit ups
✓ 7, 6, 5, all the way down to 1 push up and 1 sit up

Jog for another 5 minutes

✓ Do 10 tricep dips, then 10 bicep curls
✓ 9 tricep dips, 9 bicep curls
✓ 8, 7, 6….all the way down to 1 each

Jog for another 5 minutes

✓ Do 10 squats, 10 jumping jacks
✓ 9 squats, 9 jumping jacks
✓ 8, 7, 6…all the way down to 1 (Repeat whole cycle if you are advanced)

WALK for a cool down and stretch!

These were just a few examples; the list is endless, be creative. It will make your workout go by faster than a monotonous run on the treadmill. Keep these in mind when creating your own circuit:
Always start with a warm-up to wake up your muscles.
Include five to six multi-joint exercises that cover the whole body.
Always switch muscle groups so that no two back-to-back exercises work the same area. I always use opposing muscles; biceps then triceps, hamstrings then quadriceps.
Make a plan to perform exercises by time or by number of repetitions.
Insert 2 minutes of cardio if you want to keep your heart rate high; such as jogging or jumping rope.
Once you have a routine worked out, complete the circuit up to 4 times.

Yoga

I teach yoga at Andersen Windows Corporate Office over the lunch hour. Just about everyone in the class was brand new to yoga. They expected a break from their desk and a time to relax. I explained that yoga is all about "you and your practice" and to only pay attention to your body; if you need to adapt to an easier practice, I always give options. After the first class, they all were surprised at how much they sweat and felt "the burn," while de-stressing at the same time. They were hooked. I love how each week I have new participants comment to me after class on how this has changed their life in some way...less back-pain, better food choices, happier, calmer and much more.

I started yoga because it is known to decrease stress, but lots of other benefits started happening. Stress, bad food habits, irregular timings for food, junk food, lack of energy, and thyroid problems, could be some of the reasons resulting in weight gain. Practicing yoga can help in all of these problem areas. Yoga isn't just exercise; it is a mind-body connection. It helps us become aware of our bodies and how it feels; we become more aware of which foods nourish us and which ones makes us feel lethargic and less "alive."

Yoga is also one of the most helpful workouts for fighting stubborn fat stores, especially the ones that crop up after age 40. Science finds that yoga decreases levels of stress hormones and increases insulin sensitivity, a signal to your body to burn food as fuel rather than store it as fat.

Yoga is a mind-body exercise that can do everything from tighten your buns to change your outlook on life. Most types of yoga don't have the calorie-burning abilities of aerobic exercise. A 150-pound person will burn 150 calories in an hour of doing regular yoga, compared to 311 calories for an hour of walking at 3 mph. Yoga helps weight loss in a different way; it puts you in touch with your body the way nothing else can.

The effects are subtle, and related to yoga's mind-body aspects. Yoga creates a sense of "mindfulness;" which is the ability to monitor what is happening internally. When participants achieve this, it helps change relationships of mind to body; and in time to food and eating. Yoga forges a strong mind-body connection that ultimately helps make you more aware of what you eat and how it feels to be full. In yoga you learn your body is not your enemy, and the conscious awareness of the body that you gain translates into better appetite control. Yoga makes you more inclined to change your lifestyle; so if you are thinking you want to change your routine, the way you think about food, or you want to get over harmful eating patterns, yoga enhances a spiritual connection to your body that can help you make those changes a reality.

NUTRIENT Timing

Nutrient Timing is an interesting ground-breaking topic in the nutrition and fitness world. Conventional nutritionists help their clients figure out how many calories to eat and where those calories should come from (good carbs vs. bad carbs). But some nutritionists, like me, have also been trained in exercise science; I believe it is very important to find a nutritionist that can tie in exercise with diet; which increases our health in a variety of ways. Nutrient timing is the body's ability to tolerate certain nutrients changes during the day. Eating at specific time intervals each day, our hormones that build and repair, anabolic, can be increased while hormones that destroy or breakdown, catabolic, will be under control. But if you are like most Americans and don't exercise to the point of exhaustion, the values of nutrient timing are not going to help. Yes, glucose tolerance and insulin sensitivity are altered during the course of a day but these changes are not serious enough to determine nutritional timing. For these clients, I focus on what and how much to eat.

But, for the athlete or fitness buff nutrient timing should not be underestimated. Walking on a treadmill for 40 minutes 5 times a week doesn't mean you need to follow these meal suggestions. Nutrient timing is great for athletes, but for the other 99 percent of the world, it's probably the wrong thing. Unless your muscles are screaming from lifting extreme weights or you pushed your body to exhaustion, and you aren't hungry, don't worry about cramming food in your mouth in order to lose weight. The Journal of Applied Physiology, Nutrition and Metabolism and the Journal of Applied Physiology detail these findings. For one study, volunteers were asked to walk on a treadmill for an hour a day, burning about 500 calories each session. **Half of the group was given a high** carbohydrate drink (like chocolate milk) immediately after their workout while the other half abstained. Exercise increased insulin efficiency by 40 percent in those who did not eat afterwards. But the benefit was completely wiped out for those who had a high-carb drink after sweating.

These results had the researchers wondering if the type of calorie would make any difference. For the second study, volunteers cycled for 75 minutes. Immediately after exercising, half of the participants ate a meal high in carbohydrates while the other half ate a meal low in carbohydrates and high in protein but containing the same number of calories. The study found that the ability of insulin to clear sugar from the blood was greater among people who ate the low-carb meal. Numerous studies prove time after time that taking in carbohydrates immediately after working out blunts or diminishes the exercise benefit for fat loss.

As for athletes, science has now indisputably shown that 'nutrient timing' has huge implications for enhancing our health, body composition, and daily activities. First, science is pointing to the fact that if you exercise frequently, the body is primed for fat gain or fat loss just as it is primed for muscle gain or muscle loss during specific times of the day. If you eat the wrong foods at the wrong times you're impairing your hard work in the gym. Eat the right foods and your hard work will be enhanced.

Even if you are losing weight, "negative energy balance," and you aren't taking advantage of nutrient timing, you are more than likely losing equal amounts of fat and muscle.

There are three significant times of the day in which nutrient timing takes on a superior value. These times are known as the Energy Phase, The Anabolic Phase, and The Growth Phase. I also like to include something called The Rest of The Day Phase.

The Energy Phase is called this because this phase occurs during the workout when energy demands are highest. The energy used by skeletal muscle is ATP. This ATP is produced and re-synthesized by macronutrients from our diet; carbs, proteins, and fats contribute indirectly to the energy of muscle contraction. Eating a meal consisting of a protein and small amount of carbohydrate immediately prior to exercise can actually increase blood flow to the muscle. Protein helps us replenish our blood with amino acids and carbs increase glucose; the protein balance of the muscle will be shifted toward the positive and glycogen depletion will be significantly reduced.

Another bonus is that the amino acids and glucose can also decrease cortisol and improve the overall immune response. It is essential during the Energy Phase to ingest some protein and a small amount of carbohydrate. How much to eat really has a lot to do with how much energy you're expending during the exercise session, how much you're eating the rest of the day, and whether your main goal is to increase muscle mass or lose body fat.

The Energy Phase meal is also very important on a hormonal level, meaning that if you eat the right balance of protein and carbohydrates post workout you can manipulate these hormones naturally for an increase in growth hormone and insulin. Human growth hormone (HGH) and insulin are both vital hormones. Eating protein after a hard workout will increase the HGH, which burns fat. **Recent studies show that holding off and not eating for 30 minutes will increase HGH even further.** Eating carbohydrates will increase insulin, which in the Energy Phase will help build more muscle. I used to eat almonds (which are actually a carbohydrate) right after a kick-butt weight lifting session, but with the new science coming out, I have been waiting 30 minutes to eat a quality high-protein meal and only consuming l-glutamine right after (see supplement chapter).

The Anabolic Phase occurs immediately after the workout and lasts about an hour or two. This phase is titled "anabolic" because it's during this time that the muscle cells are ready for muscle building. Interestingly, even though our cells are prepared for muscle building, in the absence of a good nutritional plan, this phase can continue to remain catabolic. New data shows that with the right nutritional intervention we can actually restore and enhance muscle quality during and immediately after exercise. And the best part is that if we do the nutrition thing right, not only do we repair our muscles during and after exercise, we continue to alter muscle size and quality later on as well. During the Anabolic Phase it's important to eat some protein and carbohydrate. This is our most forgiving meal. Most carbohydrate ingested during and immediately after exercise will either be oxidized for fuel or sent to the muscle and liver for glycogen resynthesis and that even in the presence of increased insulin concentrations, the post-exercise period is marked by a dramatic increase in fat metabolism.

In using this strategy, carbohydrates are eaten when they will best be converted into muscle glycogen and encourage muscle growth and repair. If muscle gain is your goal, you'll get more muscle per gram of carbohydrate ingested. **If fat loss is your goal, you'll get more muscle glycogen and a definite muscle sparing effect with fewer daily carbs ingested.** And if athletic performance is your goal, your recovery will improve considerably by consuming more protein.

During the Growth Phase, the body is under construction and it's moving quickly back toward normal physiological functioning. To put it in nutrition terms, the growth window is closing and this means bye-bye to improved insulin sensitivity. You can also sit back and watch your growth hormone levels fall. Muscle protein turnover is also slowing down. At this time it is important to ditch the high glycemic carbohydrates. While carbohydrates helped build muscle during the Energy and Anabolic phases, you'll have to stop enjoying them during the Growth Phase and the "Rest of the Day" Phase. Elevated insulin during these times is a fast track to excess fat.

During the Growth Phase and the Rest of the Day Phase focus your meals on slower digesting proteins; such as meats, cottage cheese, and eggs. Eating low glycemic carbohydrates; such as low starch vegetables. The Rest of the Day is marked by normal physiology; the food you eat during this phase should be adapted to what you know about your tolerance to carbohydrates. For example, some of you may have relatively poor carbohydrate tolerance and insulin sensitivity. As a result, you should be eating mostly protein and a blend of fats during Rest of the Day. Rest of the Day Phase is what's left after your exercise and the 6 hours post-exercise. During this time, it's important to use what you know about your body to determine what to eat and your goals to determine how much to eat. Some of you can get away with a few carbohydrate and protein meals with healthy fats thrown in. Others will have to go protein and fat meals with some veggies thrown in.

1. Eat frequently - every 3-4 hours: Eating frequently can assist with better glucose tolerance, decreased insulin response to carbohydrates, decreased blood cortisol (our stress hormone that stores fat), decreased triglyceride levels, decreased body fat, and maintenance of metabolism. Eating frequently can help you control your sugar levels, control your cholesterol, decrease triglycerides and body fat...but 100 calorie snack packs every few hours isn't going to work here! We need quality real food...an organic hard-boiled egg.

2. Take advantage of post-workout fat burning: Within 1 hour after exercise, the body prioritizes fat burning while, at the same time, increases carbohydrate storage. This is a unique time as the body usually burns a mixture of carbs and fat; eating protein keeps your body burning carbs and fat. This is great news if you've got some fat to lose!

3. If you are craving dessert, use post-workout carbohydrates wisely: As a result of the body's post-exercise shift in fuel burning/storage, carbohydrates eaten during and after exercise are much less likely to provoke fat storage than they would be during the rest of the day. You won't burn as much fat, but you also won't store it either; it will build more muscle. **The take home message here is you have to earn your dessert by exercising first!** An even safer bet would be to choose one of my "healthified" desserts!

So, in the end, using nutrient timing to your advantage means, among other things, eating every 3-4 hours, saving your carb cravings for after exercise, and eating meals composed of proteins, healthy fats, and veggies the rest of the day. Using these nutrition strategies can carry you a long way toward an improved body figure.

Menstrual Cycle Timing

The menstrual cycle not only regulates fertility, it also affects the female system in many ways. Studies usually focus on men in experiments because women are on a constant change of natural chemicals that compose the menstrual cycle makes it very difficult to create correct and reliable results. This goes to show just how influential the menstrual cycle is; it affects every aspect of a woman's makeup. That includes our lean muscle mass, our ability to burn carbohydrates and our rate of perceived effort during exercise. Yet it's also found that exercise can have influential effects on the menstrual cycle; such as using exercise to limit the pain of cramps. Working out at specific times of our cycle can greatly enhance or hinder our fat-burning potential. By altering your training and diet to accommodate certain biological changes natural to the cycle, you can enhance your accomplishments in the gym, which is called "periodization." This is the "when and how" to work out to maximize your fat-burning potential. Here is the most effective way to modify our diet and workouts to help us "go with the flow."

Days 1-4: Menstruation

Most women think of this as the end of their cycle, but in medical terms, menstruation is actually considered the beginning. Estrogen and progesterone are the two main hormones involved in the menstrual cycle; which have dropped, signaling the uterus to contract and shed its lining; which can create painful cramps.

>> EXERCISE: Aerobic exercise can help combat menstrual cramps. Prostaglandins are chemicals produced during this time, causing cramps. They are produced by the endometrium (lining of the uterus) as it's being thinned. The prostaglandins promote the uterus to contract, which can limit blood flow to the uterine muscle, depriving it of oxygen therefore causing intense pain. An intense cardio session can reduce pain by dilating blood vessels, shuttling an abundant supply of oxygen to the muscles. Cardio can also help lift your spirits; it produces endorphins and boosts serotonin, the feel-good brain chemicals that are related to runner's high. Serotonin is created, in part, by healthy estrogen from our ovaries, so when it is low we often have low moods, trouble sleeping and CRAVINGS. I suggest to add half an hour of high-intensity cardio; such as running, cycling, or swimming to your exercise program on the first two days of your period along with 200mg of 5-HTP (see Supplement chapter). Repeat on days you are experiencing strong cramps.

>> NUTRITION: Magnesium Citrate or Magnesium Glycinate is a natural miracle cure for menstrual cramps. Read "The Magnesium Miracle," to discover the wide range of benefits. Try 400-800mg/day. It is

a natural muscle relaxant, so if you take it before bed, it can also help you sleep and calm those chocolate cravings. Eating foods high in zinc before the start of menstruation is also found to prevent cramps. The journal called, Medical Hypotheses, studied women taking 30 mg of zinc 1-3 times a day. Their studies found women supplementing with zinc one to four days before their period starts can relieve all cramping. Sounds worth a try to me!

Days 5-13: Follicular Phase

The follicular phase is about a week into the menstrual cycle. Menstruation ends and estrogen levels begin to rise. The ovaries have between seven and fifteen follicles in them that are triggered to mature into eggs. One egg becomes dominant and is released, while the others simply die.

>> EXERCISE: The American Journal of Physiology in 2006 examined glycogen, carbohydrate, usage in the different phases of the menstrual cycle. They consistently found that during the follicular phase, carbohydrates are burned preferentially during exercise. This means glycogen stores are used up faster than at other times of the month. This type of food energy is a great supply for high-intensity interval training (HIIT). This means bump up the intensity, which will help deplete glycogen stores and help burn more fat. This workout is when you run as fast as you can for 1 minute, then recover and walk for one minute. HIIT also enhances our resting metabolism after our workout. HITT causes an "afterburn" effect; which causes us to continue to burn calories after the workout because our muscles are repairing themselves. The "afterburn" effect boosts our fat-burning abilities.

>> NUTRITION: True, you can eat more carbohydrates during this phase of your cycle than you might normally, but it's essential to your health that the majority of your carbohydrates come from coconut flour, nuts and fibrous veggies. Make sure you are still getting your essential fatty acids; quality fats over quantity at this time.

Day 14: Ovulation

Ovulation is more of a dividing point between the follicular and luteal phases. Ovulation occurs when the prevailing egg is released from the ovary. It's joined by a large spike in estrogen levels.

Days 15-28: Luteal Phase

Instantly after ovulation, the follicle incubates then splits open to release the egg. It begins to increase progesterone; in turn makes a cozy lining in the uterus for possible implantation of an embryo. Progesterone also increases our basal body temperature and is the main guilty culprit for all the issues that come along with premenstrual syndrome; bloating, moodiness, acne, all those fun things.

>> EXERCISE: The European Journal of Applied Physiology, researchers measured metabolic indicators in a group of women who exercised at different phases in their menstrual cycles. The findings showed that women in the luteal phase had higher body temperatures, higher heart rates (about 10 beats per minute higher) and higher rates of perceived exertion, which means aerobic exercise feels harder now than in the follicular phase. The study also showed that the body relies on fat for fuel during the luteal phase. This is the best time to work out at a lower intensity but for longer periods to increase fat-burning during this phase. Women also have greater strength and are less fatigued by weight-training sessions during this phase. So increase those weights and maximize your muscles! I promise you won't end up like "The Incredible Hulk" unless you overdo the carbohydrates.

>> NUTRITION: The increase in basal body temperature during the luteal phase also increases sweat rate. Be sure to keep hydrated by drinking enough water and maintain electrolyte balance. This doesn't mean you need Gatorade...no one needs that stuff...it is filled with junk. During the luteal phase it is important to eat more fat and less carbohydrates because this is the preferred energy source. Trans-fats are still the devil...always choose good fats.

Most women will have around 480 cycles in a lifetime. Taking advantage of these hormonal changes can help us reach our peak fitness levels.

How to Burn More Calories Walking!

1. Vary the Speed.

Walking at the same pace all the time doesn't challenge your body as much as varying the speed. Instead of walking at a steady speed for thirty minutes, alternate walking a medium pace for three minutes followed by a faster pace for three minutes. The pace you choose for your second three minutes should be fast enough so that it's difficult for you to talk. During that three minutes, really focus on your movements. Alternate fast-slow intervals five times for a total workout time of thirty minutes. Not only will you burn more calories, you'll also build up endurance.

2. Take it to the Beach...or snow.

Walking on sand burns up to 50% more calories compared to walking on a smooth surface such as pavement. Take advantage of this the next time you're at the beach and you'll look even better in your bikini.

3. Wear a Weighted Vest.

You can buy weighted vests that will allow you to burn more calories while walking. If you don't want to purchase a weighted vest, strap a backpack with a few books onto your back before heading out the door. The more a person weighs the more calories they burn; therefore, using more force with the added weight will also achieve a higher calorie burn. Avoid using dumbbells or hand weights while walking since they can increase the risk of injury.

4. Get your Whole Body Involved.

When you walk, use as much of your body as you can. Keep your arms pumping through your entire workout using exaggerated movements to burn more calories.

5. Listen to music or audio book.

Put on some high energy music. Studies have shown that people exercise harder and longer when they're listening to upbeat, fast paced music. It also makes the time go by more quickly. I also find listening to a favorite podcast or book can help the time fly by!

6. Head for the Hills.

If you walk outside, change your route so you come upon a few hills to get your heart rate up and burn more fat and calories. Try to maintain the same pace going up the hill as you do on level ground. You'll burn more calories, increase endurance, and build lower body strength by adding some inclines.

7. Walk with an Energetic Dog.

An eager dog can not only motivate you, but help you burn more fat. You'll be prone to move faster when you have an enthusiastic canine by your side who absolutely craves exercise. It is an animal instinct to desire exercise.

CHAPTER 6

balance. This ha...
the stress du...
hormon...
reg...

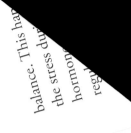

HORMONES

Hormones run our metabolism

When I start talking to clients about our hormones and our weight, they usually get a surprised look on their face. What do hormones have to do with our weight? A hormone is a chemical messenger from a cell in the body. A hormone is produced by almost every organ system and is secreted directly into the bloodstream. Hormones signal certain cells to perform certain functions. Hormones are in charge of so many important pieces of our everyday life; our monthly mood swings, sex drive, blood sugar levels, muscle tone, fat burning ability, metabolism, immune system…the list is huge! Hormones play a role in everything from good sleep and good sex to headaches, stress, fatigue and weight gain.

The struggle to lose weight can be very difficult, and many feel that there has to be a reason that the weight is not coming off. It is true that hormonal imbalance affects some overweight individuals. Hormones do play a role in weight loss and gain, but the role is dependent on the individual, and his or her dietary and exercise choices.

Hormones can affect our mood and energy amount. We, however, affect hormones. Our way of life plays a huge role in the hormonal makeup inside us. For example, if a person is inactive, certain hormones decrease, such as testosterone. Testosterone is a hormone that works to increase metabolism, and therefore regulate weight and encourage weight loss. On the other hand, a more active person will have a greater number of chemical reactions in the blood, and help enhance the body's hormonal

...ppens so the body can cope with its own need to adapt to ...ng physical exertion. As a result, the body will create balanced ...s, which boosts metabolism, and lead to weight loss. By exercising ...arly, getting adequate sleep, and eating the right foods, the body can create harmony with your hormones.

Thyroid

I like to compare the thyroid gland to cruise control in a car. Cruise control keeps a car running at a constant speed without having to keep a steady foot on the gas pedal. The thyroid hormone does the same thing; it keeps pieces in the body working at the proper speed. But problems come in if our thyroid's cruise control starts to malfunction. If thyroid hormone levels decrease, known as hypothyroidism, the rest of the body also decreases in activity. This means the cells need less energy (calories) and extra energy will be stored as fat. Weight will increase even though the appetite decreases. Often times, a person will feel cold because less heat is produced and the sweat glands no longer keep the skin moist. The brain wants to sleep all the time, the heart beats slower, the Basal Metabolic Rate slows, the bowels become sluggish. The whole body slows down.

If thyroid levels increases, it is referred to as hyperthyroidism. The body increases in activity; which means more energy (calories) are used up. Fat and protein stores are mobilized and weight decreases even though the appetite increases. Hyperthyroid patients are often hot because more heat is produced and sweating increases in an effort to cool off. The brain is in overtime; which causes irritability and shakiness. Sleep becomes difficult; which makes symptoms worse. Heart beat speeds up, bowel activity increases. The whole body speeds up.

The thyroid is not strictly necessary for life, but it does have profound effects on our body, such as metabolism, fertility, growth, development, cardiovascular and central nervous system.

1. **Metabolism**: Thyroid hormones fuel complex metabolic activities that increase our basal metabolic rate. The thyroid can cause an increase body heat production, which increases oxygen consumption and rates of ATP (energy).

Fat metabolism: Increased thyroid hormone levels boost fat mobilization; this amplifies concentrations of fatty acids in the blood. Blood concentrations of cholesterol and triglycerides are inversely connected with thyroid hormone levels; hypothyroidism is linked to high blood cholesterol levels.

Carbohydrate metabolism: Thyroid hormones fuel our body's ability to burn carbohydrates. Hypothyroidism can increase risk of diabetes because our thyroid enhances insulin-dependent entry of glucose into cells to generate free glucose. When our thyroid is sluggish, we start to become insulin resistant.

2. **Reproductive system:** The thyroid hormone controls our sex hormones. Hypothyroidism is frequently associated with infertility.

3. **Growth:** Thyroid hormones are necessary for normal growth. Thyroid deficiencies in children results in growth retardation. The human growth hormone and the thyroid hormones are intimately connected.

4. **Development:** An experiment on tadpoles demonstrates the effects of the thyroid and development. The tadpoles were deprived thyroid hormones; which resulted in an inability to endure metamorphosis into frogs. Thyroid hormones are vital for fetal and neonatal brain development.

5. **Cardiovascular system:** Thyroid hormones controls heart rate, contractility and cardiac output. It also supports blood flow to many organs.

6. **Central nervous system:** The thyroid hormones control our mental state. Hypothyroid patients often feel mentally sluggish, while hyperthyroid patience often feel anxious and irritable.

BALANCE YOUR THYROID LEVELS

Our thyroid runs so many pieces of our body. Following a few diets and lifestyle changes can help regulate our thyroid output. Some foods can aggravate existing thyroid issues; such as cruciferous veggies, which have enzymes that interfere with thyroid output. Sleep and exercise, specifically yoga, can be very therapeutic for our thyroid.

Ways to support the thyroid:	What Happens:	Sources:
Fish	Fatty fish are great sources of iodine and omega-3s, both enhance thyroid functions.	Try salmon, herring, sardines, or anchovies. If you don't care for fish, an omega 3 supplement can be very helpful.
Coconut Oil	Healthy fats are essential to a proper running thyroid.	Choose healthy fats like coconut oil, macadamia nut oil, and nuts. I make all of my baked goods with coconut oil.
Iodine	Iodine is essential for a healthy thyroid.	Using "SEA SALT" is stripped of iodine, make sure to buy mineralized sea salt. I also recommend a Kelp supplement.
Selenium	Selenium assists our thyroid by converting thyroxine (T) to the active form (T3).	Add in brazil nuts and brewer's yeast. A quality multivitamin can also help.
Zinc	Zinc encourages the pituitary gland to release TSH.	Don't be afraid of red meat, which is filled with zinc. Other sources are lamb, sesame and pumpkin seeds, and spinach.
Exercise and Yoga	Thyroxine is a hormone released by the thyroid that raises our basal metabolic rate. This hormone is increased over 30% during exercise and stays high for hours afterward.	Get your heart pumping by walking, running, swimming…. Yoga also massages the endocrine system which regulates thyroid output.

Ways to deplete the thyroid:	What Happens:	Sources:
Caffeine	Caffeine over stimulates the adrenals, which aggravates thyroid issues.	If you need a little pick-me-up, choose green tea; which has caffeine, but it also has l-theanine to off-set the caffeine stimulation. Keep coffee, black tea, chocolate, caffeinated soda to a minimum.
Cruciferous veggies	These foods can interfere with thyroid medications. Isothiocyanates in cruciferous veggies upset normal cellular communications in the thyroid.	Always cook cruciferous veggies: broccoli, cauliflower, kale, collard greens, spinach, and Brussels sprouts to lower the enzymes that interfere with our thyroid output.
Goitrogenic foods	These foods inhibit the thyroid to use iodine, which is essential for the thyroid.	Watch out for peaches, peanuts, strawberries, pine nuts, and bamboo shoots.
Refined Carbohydrates	Simple carbohydrates cause a surge then abrupt drop in blood sugar levels; which decrease energy levels even further.	Stay away from sugar, baked goods, ice cream, white rice, pasta, bread, refined grains, potatoes, and corn.
Soy	Soy isoflavones may reduce thyroid levels by inhibiting important enzymes.	Steer clear from concentrated amounts of soy; such as faux meat products, soy milk, or soy butter. Pure forms of soy like tempeh are fine in moderation.
Inadequate Sleep	Sleep deprivation lowers secretion of the thyroid hormones.	Aim for 8 hours of quality sleep every night.

Glucagon and insulin connection

I'd like to introduce you to an awesome fat-burning hormone called glucagon. Don't confuse this with glycogen. Glycogen is stored sugar in the muscles and liver; increasing insulin. Glucagon is the opposite hormone to insulin. Insulin takes sugars and carbohydrates you eat and stores it as fat. Glucagon takes the stored fat and breaks it down into sugar, creating a "fat burning" response. Do I have you intrigued?

In the presence of insulin, you can't burn fat for energy. Eating the typical American diet of sugar, fat-free and refined carbohydrates stops fat burning. Overeating of any food will also increase insulin. Not only does this prevent fat burning, it also activates the storage of fat to make triglycerides and increasing LDL cholesterol. The misconception many people have is thinking all their cholesterol problems come from eating fats and cholesterol. It's the carbohydrates that cause inflammation which increases health problems of all sorts.

People wonder why I never suggest fat-free foods. Well, adding fat to your meal can actually slow the insulin response. If you added butter to your bread, it would cause less insulin response than eating the bread alone. Even ice cream with all its fat is less harmful to our waistline than eating the pure sugar alone, but I'm not recommending this.

With blood sugar imbalances, mood is easily affected. High blood sugar levels cause fatigue and brain fog, like after a Thanksgiving meal. On the flip side, too low blood sugar levels can make you feel irritable, depressed, moody, or worried, which you may have felt an hour after eating candy or after skipping a meal.

Conversely, when glucagon is stimulated, you will burn fat. There are several actions you can take to release this hormone. The first is eating adequate amounts of protein. This is why many of the high-protein diets work for people. There is a catch though, if you have liver damage or consume a lot of alcohol; which is a fat-storing carbohydrate anyway, your body can't burn protein efficiently. Glucagon works inside the liver so for a person who has a healthy liver, eating protein is fat-burning and consuming carbohydrate is fat-storing.

Glucagon is also stimulated with exercise. Exercise increases glucagon up to 5 times our normal amounts! If you combine both exercise and increase amounts of protein, you can strategically enhance your weight loss. Exercise also decreases insulin levels.

Initially, low-calorie starvation diets increase glucagon too. Which is why people lose some weight by not eating, but here are a few problems that come into play here. Not only are you losing a lot of fat-burning muscle, the hormone cortisol is also increased, which slows metabolism, releases extra sugar in the blood causing insulin to store fat in our belly, and causes a desire to grab comfort carbohydrates.

BALANCE YOUR GLUCAGONAND INSULINLEVELS

There are many ways to increase glucagon and decrease insulin. The way we eat, what we eat and how we exercise is essential to these two main hormones! Also check out Chapter 9 for "13 Tasty Substitutes that Help our Waist Line and Blood Sugar Levels" for more food tips.

Increase Glucagon and Decrease Insulin With:	What Happens:	Sources :
Protein	Begin with a protein "appetizer" 10 minutes before each meal. This sends your body the right signals not to overeat, since protein stimulates the production of this appetite-regulating hormone.	Have string cheese or a small whey protein shake before you sit down to dine. Eat small amounts of protein in between meals to prevent hunger. Supplementing with amino acids help also.
Fiber	Fiber slows insulin spikes.	Get your fiber from non-starchy vegetables, psyllium husks and coconut flour.

Increase Glucagon and Decrease Insulin With:	What Happens:	Sources :
Frequent small meals	Eating small meals throughout the day keeps glucagon firing… which means more fat burning.	This doesn't mean a 100 calorie snack-pack every 2 hours. Always include a protein at meals and snacks; such as hard-boiled eggs, string cheese, or a handful of almonds.
Exercise	Glucagon breaks down fat so that it can be used as fuel. Glucagon typically begins to be secreted after 30 minutes of exercise when blood glucose levels begin to be depleted.	If fat loss is your goal, exercise in the morning on an empty stomach so glucagon doesn't have to wait for glucose to be depleted. If you must eat something before your workout, try a hard-boiled egg or coconut oil.
Choose vegetables for your carbohydrates	Vegetables also have much more potassium than sodium, which gets rid of water retention and water weight.	Increasing fiber helps hormone balance tremendously, but stay away from cereals and grains. Choose non-starchy vegetables. Leafy greens have a ton of fiber which barely increases insulin. Choosing vegetables as a carbohydrate will reduce rather than increase weight.

Decrease Glucagon and Increase Insulin With:	What Happens:	Sources:
Stress	Stress can increase cortisol; which will also increase insulin and decrease glucagon.	If you are feeling overwhelmed, find an activity, rather than comfort food to calm you. Get a massage, take a walk around a lake…just don't reach for a cookie!
Simple Carbohydrates	Carbohydrates trigger insulin; which is our fat storing hormone.	Avoid sweets and refined carbohydrates, including juice, alcohol and hidden sugars; such as ketchup, marinara sauces, salad dressings, flavored yogurt, rice cakes and even most deli meats contain sugar so check labels! Also avoid juice cleanses.
Overeating	Overeating increases insulin and decreases glucagon.	Stick with small balanced meals throughout the day.
High Sugar Fruits	Fruits sweetness comes from fructose. Fructose doesn't register our hormones to produce a "satisfied" feeling.	Always match a protein and a fat with fruit. For example; a ½ an apple with 3 tablespoons of almond butter…or ½ cup of berries on top of cottage cheese.

If you have read any of Suzanne Somers' books, you already have read about the amazing properties of human growth hormone. She is a huge advocate increasing this hormone and injects it into her body every night. I also believe that we need to increase this awesome hormone, but unlike Susan, I will tell you how to boost it through diet and exercise...which come with no scary side effects.

Human growth hormone, also known as HGH, is an amazing hormone that is produced by the pituitary gland in the brain. This hormone stimulates cell production and is responsible for increasing height, building muscle mass, keeping bones healthy, controlling sugar and insulin levels, absorption of calcium, reducing fat as well as helping numerous other functions that are fundamental for growth.

The human growth hormone is produced at full-speed when we are young but the pituitary gland slows down the production as the body ages; usually around age 30 it really starts to decline. The level of HGH peaks during puberty when there is a growth spurt. The levels continue to decline throughout our adult life. This decrease in the levels of HGH is what causes elasticity loss in our skin...wrinkles, increase issues with diabetes, depression, loss of energy, and loss of muscle mass. Increasing the levels of human growth hormone can make you look young and feel healthy.

Diet, exercise and sleep patterns all play a role in human growth hormone secretion. This hormone regulates a lot of important physiological functions, including water and energy balance, reproductive activity and controls other glands in the body. Human growth hormone is also involved in important processes that control metabolism throughout our life, including the amount of muscle, bone and collagen, the regulation of fat burning and the preservation of a healthier body composition. There is no doubt that increasing the secretion of natural human growth hormone is favorable to everyone, including those with joint pain, diabetes, blood sugar imbalances, arthritis, abnormal heart growth, muscle weakness, and increased triglycerides.

A recent discovery found that some people can have a growth hormone deficiency, which has proven just how important this hormone is. People with a deficiency have a considerably low muscle mass and high body fat; most were obese and had an increased risk of heart disease and a reduced ability to exercise.

In healthy bodies, human growth hormone secretion follows a circadian rhythm and is released in 6-12 distinct portions per day, with the largest portion secreted about an hour after the onset of night-time sleep. This is why I stress the importance of sleep! The release of human growth hormone can be triggered by a number of natural stimuli, the most powerful of which are sleep and exercise.

We just learned that the major human growth hormone surge usually happens around one hour after the onset of sleep, it is imperative for everyone, athletes most of all, to get plenty of it. Most Olympic athletes get around 10 hours of sleep a night and a 1 hour nap a day! If the quality of sleep is insufficient there will be a decline in the amount of human growth hormone released, with negative consequences for our overall physical and mental health. Significant prerequisites for good quality sleep and optimal human growth hormone secretion during sleep include a cool, dark room and a quality diet containing sufficient protein. Sleep is necessary for good health in general, and for most people this means around eight hours.

Specific exercise routines and nutritional strategies can enhance our natural secretion of HGH. There is no need to inject dangerous unnatural hormones to achieve higher levels; we just need to work to receive these safe benefits. Various studies find that HGH is triggered by exercise-induced increases in adrenaline, nitric oxide, lactate acid, and nerve activity. To achieve a surge of HGH with exercise, you need to spend at least 10 minutes working above lactate threshold intensity. This means you will be sweating and feeling the "burn." This will result in a major surge of human growth hormone secreted, with levels declining gradually over a period of an hour.

It is also known that multiple daily workouts can give a boost to optimal HGH secretion over a 24-hour period. That is why I suggest breaking up your exercise into two smaller, yet harder workout times throughout your day.

As far as diet is concerned, athletes are normally pushed to eat a diet high in carbohydrates, consuming foods with a higher glycemic index around intense exercise and starchy carbohydrates at other times of the day.

And the standard advice for fluids is to drink carbohydrate-electrolyte drinks before, during and after exercise. But, high-carb diets switch off human growth hormone secretion. **Carbo loading after exercise is not a good strategy for increasing the secretion of human growth hormone. Foods high in carbohydrates stimulate insulin release which, in turn, contributes to a reduction in human growth hormone. Americans are the only athletes that encourage the "carb loading" theory. The 2008 Kenyan Olympic marathon winner ate a huge steak with broccoli for his pre-race meal...not a plate of pasta and his lips have never touched a bottle of Gatorade!**

Hydration is also a huge piece of keeping that human growth hormone firing. Drink plenty of water during exercise is extremely important because dehydration has been found to drastically reduce the exercise-induced HGH response.

There are also a few nutritional supplements called amino acids that can increase the secretion of this youthful hormone. Amino acids come from protein and are the building blocks of our muscles. Before exercise it has been shown that intake of 1.5g of arginine will increase human growth hormone secretion. Also, consuming 2g of glutamine after exercise will boost your secretion without any side effects. It may also be a good idea to ingest a combination of amino acids after exercise; this has also been found to enhance human growth hormone secretion. I often drink a whey protein shake immediately after an intense workout; which contains high amounts of amino acids.

A high level of human growth hormone keeps body fat down and muscle mass high. The benefits are clear, so if you are intrigued, here are some suggestions of exercises and dietary strategies for optimizing your human growth hormone capabilities:

1. Exercise – aim for at least 4 sessions per week, each involving at least 10 minutes' work above lactate threshold, making sure you feel the burn!
2. Before exercise – No food, 1.5 g arginine, 2g glutamine
3. During exercise – plenty of water , NOT Gatorade
4. After exercise – avoid sugar but take 25g protein 30 minutes afterwards in the form of a protein shake, protein bar, lean meat, eggs, or cottage cheese. I prefer to take l-glutamine and arginine supplements immediately after exercise if I can't eat right away.

Our human growth hormone is responsible for our youthful physique and well-being. Natural methods of enhancing this hormone can reap a multitude of benefits. Sticking with the right foods and activities is a safe and effective way to increase this hormone without the scary use of unnatural injections.

Increase HGH with:	What they do:	Sources:
Glutamine	The amino acid glutamine is extremely helpful in boosting the immune system, aiding absorption in the intestines, and regulating the conversion of protein to muscle. L-glutamine also stimulates human growth hormone production.	Take 1-2 grams of l-glutamine after intense exercise, one hour before eating (to assist in healthy digestion), and 1 gram before bed.
Protein, Protein, Protein!	Along with exercise and sleep, protein is needed to provide the essential amino acids necessary for HGH synthesis. Protein is used by the growth hormones to build muscles.	I include whey protein in many of my baked goods to help repair my muscles and increase HGH. I love my cinnamon roll recipe with whey protein!
Arginine	The amino acids arginine and ornithine cause the pituitary gland to produce growth hormone, but only on an empty stomach. Insulin and HGH can't be present at the same time and insulin will always win.	Choose quality amino acid supplements. Start by taking two to four grams of arginine or ornithine before bed on an empty stomach.
Magnesium and Zinc	Zinc helps optimize the natural secretion of HGH and magnesium helps promote relaxation, a combination of these two minerals before sleep offers a double benefit.	Take 450mg of Magnesium Glycinate and 30mg of Zinc 30 minutes before bed to stimulate the secretion of HGH enhancing growth and regeneration of our muscles.

Increase HGH with:	What they do:	Sources:
GABA	GABA is an amino acid neurotransmitter that signals the pituitary to release HGH.	As little as 2 grams of GABA taken immediately before bed promotes the development of lean tissue while decreasing body fat.
Potassium	A potassium deficiency has been found to cause growth hormone suppression.	Animal protein, greens, Avocado, Fish, and spinach are all rich in potassium.
Water	Scientists have discovered that cell volume regulates cell function. Hormones and nutrients are best utilized when we are properly hydrated.	Water, water, water! 95% of our culture is chronically dehydrated!
Going to bed on an empty stomach.	Studies show that HGH is significantly higher if the body is fasting before sleep.	Don't eat 3 hours before bed, in particular stay away from carbohydrates…sorry no popcorn with your movie!
Sleep	HGH is very dependent on sleep because a major surge occurs 30-70 minutes after falling asleep. Disturbed or interrupted sleep can cause HGH output to be reduced or eliminated.	Aim for 7-9 uninterrupted hours a night.
Intense Exercise	Vigorous weight training has been proven to increase HGH. The more aggressive and intense the workout, the more HGH is released.	Make sure your muscles are screaming at the end of your workout! A leisure walk around the block won't help you here.

Decrease HGH with:	What they do:	Sources:
Eating before bed...	Eating too close to bedtime raises your body temperature, increases blood sugar and insulin, prevents the release of melatonin and diminishes the release of HGH.	Eating any food, in particular those filled with carbohydrates... I included this again because it is very important!!!
Sodium	Cellular dehydration and shrinkage has been strongly linked to many diseases and is essential in maintaining a healthy cell structure. By **increasing your potassium** intake and **reducing your sodium intake**, you shift water from the outer parts of your cells into them.	Potassium levels decline with age, as does HGH. Increase your water intake and be aware of the sodium in foods. Also increase potassium to flush out excess sodium.
Carbohydrates	HGH and insulin cannot both exist in the blood stream. When high carb foods are eaten, insulin wins and HGH is eliminated.	Stay away from refined carbohydrates during times when your body produces more human growth hormone, such as after intense exercise or before bed.
Stress	Our body's response to stress is a rise in cortisol, the catabolic, pro-aging, anti-immunity, anti-testosterone, anti-growth hormone, insulin-raising hormone.	Cortisol breaks down muscle tissue, indirectly promotes a buildup of belly fat, and interferes with quality sleep.

Did you ever wonder why it is easier to gain weight as compared to keeping it off? The key to this is in the fat cells where a powerful hormone is produced called leptin. Leptin signals the brain to regulate the metabolism in order to store or to burn fat.

Research shows that an estimate of over 85% of people who had lost weight, end up regaining weight because the "metabolic thermostat" of the body, leptin, is reset upward automatically. When people lose weight, leptin production decreases, which causes people to regain the lost weight. This protein hormone is derived from fat cells so when you lose fat, leptin levels drop. When you gain fat, leptin levels rise. Once leptin is secreted by your fat cells, it travels to the hypothalamus; which controls eating behavior. Once it's there, leptin activates anorectic nerve cells, which decreases your appetite. At the same time, leptin stops cells from stimulating your appetite. To put it simply, when leptin levels drop, you get hungry. When they go up, you feel full.

As well as being affected by total body fat levels, leptin levels will rise and fall quite rapidly in response to both overfeeding and underfeeding. After the initial drop in response to underfeeding, leptin declines at a rate that's linked more closely to the loss of fat.

Some scientists refer to leptin as an "anti-obesity hormone," but it is now being called an "anti-starvation" hormone because it tells our brains what to do when our fat stores are in short supply.

To demonstrate the power of leptin, scientists gave leptin injections to lean and obese volunteers who had recently lost weight. The team found that most of the metabolic and hormonal changes were reversed once leptin levels were restored to pre-weight loss levels; which means the volunteers had a hard time keeping the weight from creeping back on. In the study, subjects were fed 800 calories per day until they'd lost 10% of their weight. This led to a drop in both leptin and thyroid hormone concentrations, along with a reduction in the metabolic rate. For the next five weeks, subjects received low-dose leptin injections twice a day to bring leptin back to pre-diet levels. These injections of leptin reversed the drop in energy expenditure and increased thyroid hormone levels. The participants also continued to lose fat while conserving muscle tissue.

Another impact is that a drop in leptin concentrations seems to play a bigger part on your body than increasing leptin levels above the normal physiological range. The primary functional role of leptin is to defend, not reduce, body fat by increasing appetite and decrease energy expenditure when fat stores are low. Physiological responses to levels of leptin below and above this threshold is very unbalanced; low levels of leptin triggers a strong counter-regulation to a "perceived" threat to survival; levels of leptin above the threshold signals a "sufficient" or excess fat stores are not responded to. In other words, your body will have to fight harder against losing fat than it will against gaining fat. That's why most people find it a whole lot easier to get fat than they do to get lean.

Unfortunately, there is no easy route of just taking a leptin pill to help solve our weight problems. First of all, leptin can't be taken orally because our stomach can't absorb it. Leptin needs to be injected for it to be absorbed; every day; for life! This is both inconvenient and very expensive.

A more practical and healthy solution is to follow a diet of cycling your calorie and carbohydrate intake throughout the course of a week. A day of controlled overeating will raise leptin levels and can help you avoid some of the metabolic adaptations natural with any type of restricted-calorie diet. I'm not talking about a full blown "cheat day;" not like you are thinking anyway. Full blown "cheat days" have the ability to undo all of the hard work you've done during the previous six days.

Instead, people who are restricting calories can profit from a kind of planned break during the week. By having one free meal or throughout the day increase your total calories appropriately with each meal can help with leptin. Your choice will depend on how low your calorie intake is, how lean you are, and your rate of fat loss.

LEPTIN RESISTANCE

So after all this information, you'd think that having extra fat stores create more leptin, but that is where an interesting mystery comes into play. 98 percent of those who are significantly overweight are leptin-resistant. Most defects in leptin signaling may lead to obesity, overeating and less energy expenditure. Leptin-resistance is similar to insulin-resistance in that it occurs after being overexposed to high levels of the hormone. At this point, the body no longer responds to the hormone. Much like high blood sugar levels result in surges in insulin, sugar metabolized in fat cells causes the fat to release surges in leptin. Over time, leptin-resistance may develop.

The best way to reduce your chances of diabetes is to avoid surges in leptin; which is the leading cause of leptin-resistance. Eating the typical American diet, full of refined sugars and other processed foods, is a guaranteed way to cause undesired surges. Focusing your diet on simple, unprocessed real foods like vegetables is currently the best way to prevent leptin-resistance.

BALANCE YOUR LEPTIN LEVELS

To recap, after you eat, your body releases leptin; which tells your body to stop feeling hungry and start burning calories. An interesting paradox is that the more fat your body carries, the more leptin you produce, but your body starts to become resistant; a lot like insulin resistance. The objective is to optimize your levels of this hormone by eating foods that increase your body's sensitivity to leptin and eating foods that work with other hormones to regulate leptin's functions.

Increase Leptin With:	What Happens:	Sources:
Fish	Eating fish can help by changing the way your body responds to leptin. Although leptin levels are usually lower in women, the researchers found the leptin levels of women who ate fish to be twice as high of both female and male vegetarians.	Choose fish filled with omega 3's; such as salmon and tuna.
Protein	Protein improves leptin sensitivity, which lowers calorie intake by helping you feel full faster.	Increasing your protein to at least 30 grams for breakfast and at least another 60 throughout the day. Choose quality proteins like salmon and pasture eggs. A whey protein smoothie in the morning is a great leptin stabilizer!
Omega-3s	Eating omega-3 fatty acids may cause a brief dip in leptin levels and give it the boost you are looking for.	Choose foods rich in omega-3s like salmon, flaxseeds, walnut oil, walnuts, and organic eggs. A supplement can also do the trick.
EPA (an omega-3)	EPA increases leptin production by enhancing the metabolism of glucose.	Cold-water fish, wild salmon, mackerel, sardines, and herring.
Zinc	Zinc increases leptin levels.	Oysters have the most zinc per serving than any other food. Chicken and red meat also provide the lots of zinc. Other sources include nuts, and seafood.

Decrease Leptin With:	What Happens:	Sources:
A large dinner	Eating all you calories at dinner delays leptin production for 2 hours after the meal.	Never starve yourself all day just to consume all your calories at night, constantly eating small meals optimize the release of leptin.
Alcohol	The body takes the leptin away with the alcohol into the liver.	Keep alcohol consumption to a minimum.
Caffeine	Consuming lots of caffeine lowers leptin levels. Caffeine does increase metabolism, but it also can mess with a lot of our hormones.	Keep caffeine consumption to around 300 mg if you are trying to lose weight.
Fructose	Fructose is an interesting sweetener. We need insulin to tell our body to produce leptin, but unlike other sweeteners, fructose doesn't stimulate insulin, and therefore the body doesn't stimulate leptin. High fructose corn syrup consumption causes leptin resistance.	Soda and candy, and any food that includes the ingredient: high-fructose corn syrup (HFCS) linked to diabetes and high cholesterol. Beware…it's in everything! Ketchup, marinara sauce, baby formula…Yikes! This is also why you never want to eat fruit by itself; always include a fat and protein.
Simple Carbohydrates	Carbohydrates slow down the movement of leptin across the blood-brain barrier.	Reduce simple carbohydrates in your diet…white rice, white bread, cereals, baked goods, sugar.

Increase Leptin With:	What Happens:	Sources:
Neurotoxins	Neurotoxins cause inflammation which affects hormones. People with high toxic levels will not lose weight, regardless of diet or exercise, unless this issue is addressed.	Avoid heavy metals like mercury and lead. Also stay away from biotoxins like mold and lyme. These toxic items enter the body and attach to fat and nerve cells.

Ghrelin

Scientists believe they have discovered why people get hungry at mealtimes, why dieters who lose weight often gain it back, and why stomach surgery helps obese people lose a great deal of weight. One main reason is the hormone called ghrelin, which makes us hungry, slows metabolism, and decreases the body's ability to burn fat.

Ghrelin levels increase before meals and drop afterward. Volunteers given ghrelin injections felt extremely hungry, and, when turned loose at a buffet, ate 30 percent more than they did previously. Dieters who lose weight produce more ghrelin than they did before dieting, as if their bodies are fighting against starvation. By contrast, obese people who have gastric bypass surgery to lose weight end up with low levels of ghrelin, which helps explain why their appetites decrease noticeably after the surgery.

People who fail to sleep properly over-stimulate their ghrelin production which increases the desire for food. Lack of sleep also reduces the production of leptin which is the body's appetite suppressant. So in short, if you don't get enough sleep, the hormones in your body get all out of whack and you think that you're hungry when really you don't need that food.

Getting the right amount of sleep can be the first step to making sure that you're getting the ghrelin and leptin balance that your body needs to naturally maintain a healthy weight. Getting 8 hours of quality sleep every night will help you naturally balance out your ghrelin and leptin levels …not making up for it on the weekends. I say "quality" because many people suffer from sleep apnea and don't know it. If you have been told you snore, kick, talk, or stop breathing in the night, have your doctor check for sleep apnea. Sleep disorders will keep you from getting into REM sleep which is when our hormones are balanced. Allergies are a main cause of sleep apnea…you don't have to be overweight to suffer from it.

This information has helped scientists harness information to assist people in losing weight. Scientists have created an anti-obesity vaccine which reduces the production of ghrelin which helps reduce cravings. Yes, these drugs are on the market, but instead of putting a huge dent in your wallet, you can start to balance ghrelin by following a few easy steps.

BALANCE YOUR GHRELIN LEVELS

Ghrelin creates our ravenous cravings for food. Our bodies increase this hormone before eating, whether it is when your clock strikes 12noon at work or you walk by a bakery and the smell of doughnuts stimulates the production. Follow these steps to keep your ghrelin levels in check.

Decrease Ghrelin With:	What Happens:	Sources
Eating at the same time	Scientists have discovered that ghrelin levels rise and fall at your usual mealtimes; eating on a schedule prevents over-production of ghrelin.	Always keep an emergency pack in your car or bag to keep the ghrelin spikes at bay. I always keep almonds and "healthified" protein muffin with me.
Breakfast	Eating a large breakfast produces 33% less ghrelin throughout the day. People also feel more satisfied for longer periods of time.	Have a quality breakfast every morning like an omelet with veggies.
Fiber	Fiber helps keep ghrelin levels down.	Use coconut flour, psyllium husks and almond flour for baked goods!
Low-calorie, high-volume foods	Ghrelin remains high until the stomach feels the food touching the sides. Filling your belly with low-calorie, high-volume foods keep ghrelin levels at bay.	Non-starchy veggies are your best bet. Eat veggies that have a high water content. This is why eating a salad or a bowl of broth-based soup helps you eat less.
Protein	Protein suppresses ghrelin. Whey protein is the best protein at keeping hunger pains away.	Choose quality whey protein with no sugar; like Jay Robb. Eating the protein portion in a meal before your starch also helps decrease ghrelin faster.

Increase Ghrelin With:	What Happens:	Sources:
Crispy, high carb foods	Carbohydrates lower ghrelin fast, but for a short period of time; on the other hand, protein lowers ghrelin slower, but for a longer time.	French fries, potato chips, deep-fried foods…did I really need to tell you these are bad?
Smelling doughnuts at work!	Just by smelling certain foods tells your brain to increase ghrelin. Your body anticipates the sweet sinful foods and actually prepares for the first bite.	Stay away from foods that create a binge. If you need to, take a different route to work to avoid those tempting bakeries.
Eating before bed	Eating before bed increases ghrelin levels; which inhibits quality sleep. Keeping your ghrelin levels low will help induce sleep.	Try not to eat 3 hours before bed.
Excessive dieting	Don't skip meals. This causes a dramatic increase in ghrelin levels…up to 24%.	Be patient with weight loss, skipping meals and reverting to meal-replacement drinks is a short-lived way to losing weight. Going too low in calories creates an insatiable appetite.
Fructose	Fructose, a type of sugar, doesn't register in our body to increase insulin, which means that ghrelin will increase shortly after consumption.	Fructose is found in fruit and high-fructose corn syrup. Stay away from high fructose corn syrup and always eat fruit with a protein and fat…an apple with peanut butter.

Estrogen and Progesterone connection

Estrogen and Progesterone are powerful hormones that balance our moods, temperature, menstrual cycle, cravings, fat burning, fat storage and much more. Female problems are on the rise. Around 60% of women suffer from PMS. In addition, women suffer from an excess of hormonal imbalance symptoms, some menopausal and others not. There is strong evidence that the proper hormonal balance necessary for women's bodies to function healthily is being interfered with by a number of factors, nutrition is one of them.

Research has shown that many women in their 30s, and some even younger, will sporadically not ovulate. Without ovulation, no corpus luteum results and no progesterone is made. A progesterone deficiency occurs and several problems can happen from this, one being the month-long occurrence of unopposed estrogen which comes with lots of side-effects.

A second major problem resulting from the imbalance is the link between progesterone loss and stress. Stress along with a bad diet can provoke cycles where ovulation does not occur. The consequent lack of progesterone slows the production of the stress-busting hormones, aggravating stressful conditions that give rise to further anovulatory months and so continues the unhealthy cycle.

Estrogen's role in osteoporosis is only a minor one. Estrogen replacement will reduce bone breakdown, but only progesterone can increase new bone growth. Progesterone deficiency results in bone loss. In a three year study of 63 post-menopausal women with osteoporosis, women using topical progesterone cream experienced an average of 8% bone mass density increase in the first year, 5% the second year, and 4% in the third year. Untreated women in this age category typically lose 1.5% bone mass density per year. The use of natural progesterone along with dietary and lifestyle changes can not only stop osteoporosis but can actually reverse it, no matter what your age.

A new discovery in science now links a surprising factor to this estrogen and progesterone imbalance. The industrialized world we now live in is filled with something called petrochemical derivatives. They are in the air, food and water and include pesticides and herbicides; such as DDT, as well as various plastics found in babies bottles and water jugs, and PCBs. These chemicals mimic estrogen and are highly fat-soluble, not biodegradable or well excreted from our body, and gather in our fat tissues.

These chemicals have a mysterious ability to mimic natural estrogen and therefore are called "xeno-estrogens." Even though they are foreign chemicals, they are gathered up by the estrogen receptor sites in our body, seriously interfering with natural biochemical activity. Drinking sodas out of plastic bottles is one of the leading causes of estrogen dominance.

Extensive research is now revealing an alarming situation worldwide, effects such as reduced sperm production, cell division and sculpting of the developing brain. These "xeno-estrogens" are linked to the new discovery that sperm counts worldwide have plunged by 50% between 1938 and 1990 and also linked to genital deformities, breast, prostate and testicular cancer, and neurological disorders.

Frustrating Problems of Estrogen Dominance:
Increase in Allergies• Breast cancer • Breast tenderness • Cold hands and feet • Decreased sex drive • Mood swings • Dry eyes • Depression, anxiety, irritability • Fatigue • Fibrocystic breasts • Increase risk of strokes • Irregular periods • Headaches • Hypoglycemia • Insomnia • Slow metabolism • Infertility • PMS • Zinc deficiency • Osteoporosis • Uterine fibroids • Water retention • Weight gain • Hair loss • Acceleration of the aging • Fat gain around hips and thighs • Polycystic ovaries • Endometrial cancer • Memory loss • Thyroid dysfunction • Magnesium deficiency • Gallbladder disease • Unstable blood sugar • Cervical dysplasia • Uterine, Prostate or Ovarian cancer

Doctors have a consistent theme in women coming into the office; complaints of the uncomfortable symptoms of PMS, peri-menopause and menopause. The effects come from too much estrogen or, also known as estrogen dominance. Instead of estrogen playing its essential role within the well-balanced system of steroid hormones in our body, it has begun to overshadow the other pieces, creating a biochemical conflict.

EFFECTS OF ESTROGEN DOMINANCE

1. Excess estrogen usually means a progesterone deficiency. This deficiency leads to a decrease of new bone formation. Progesterone deficiency his is the main cause of osteoporosis.

2. When estrogen surpasses levels of progesterone, it can hinder fat burning even with hard workouts and increase weight gain. It causes headaches, irritability, chronic fatigue and loss of interest in sex. These effects are also clinically recognized as premenstrual syndrome when our estrogen is naturally higher during our menstrual cycle...now it is happening for a whole month!

3. It's been well-known that estrogen dominance promotes the development of breast cancer, but it also triggers breast tissue and can cause fibrocystic breast disease; this can be fixed by adding natural progesterone to balance the estrogen.

4. Estrogen dominance increases the risk of fibroids. One of the interesting facts about fibroids is that, regardless of the size, fibroids commonly deteriorate once menopause arrives and a woman's ovaries are no longer making estrogen.

5. Endometrial cancer can develop when estrogen dominance occurs.

Menopause and Weight Gain

It is common for estrogen levels to decrease during menopause causing a halt of ovulation. The decreased production of estrogen by the ovaries causes a woman's body to search for other sources of estrogen. Fat cells also produce estrogen, so your body learns to convert calories into fat, in order to increase estrogen production. This means weight gain.

It is also common for progesterone levels to decrease during menopause. Progesterone's role in weight gain is more deceiving; low levels of the hormone do not actually cause you to gain weight, but instead cause water retention or bloating. This annoying side effect makes you feel heavier and makes your clothes fit tighter.

6. High blood pressure and hypertension is another scary side effect of estrogen dominance. This happens because there is water retention in the cells and an increase in intercellular sodium.

7. Heart disease and strokes are connected to women who have too much estrogen.

The connection between what we put into our mouth and balancing our hormones is huge. Certain foods can decrease and increase estrogen in our body. Carbohydrates and refined sugars increase our insulin levels; which directly correlates to an increase in estrogen. Many women always ask me why I use the "full-fat" version of foods…this is one reason. Fat-free foods are replacing fats with more carbohydrates…we get enough of those without even thinking about it. We need to balance our insulin levels out with some healthy fats and proteins. Besides the real thing tastes WAY better!

BALANCE YOUR ESTROGEN AND PROGESTERONE LEVELS

Foods that impact your estrogen levels should be taken seriously. Depending on our stage in life we want to be aware of increasing or decreasing our estrogen and progesterone levels. Remember estrogen and progesterone work together. Some foods can mimic estrogen in our body; they are called phytoestrogens. During peri-menopause, phytoestrogens can help women handle the uncomfortable side effects, such as hot flashes. But during most periods in our lives, we want to limit the amount of extra estrogen in our body. Men also want to be aware of extra estrogen; some phytoestrogens can help protect your heart, but too much will decrease testosterone levels and increase risk of prostate cancer.

Decrease Estrogen With:	What Happens:	Sources:
Fiber	Estrogen is normally taken from the blood in the liver, which sends it through a tiny hole, called the bile duct, into the intestines. There, fiber soaks up estrogen and takes it out with other waste. The more fiber in our diets increases the amount of estrogen carried out.	Vegetables, coconut flour, psyllium husks and almond flour are sources of fiber. Soluble fiber is especially important. If your diet is low in fiber gradually build up tolerance to fiber along with additional water. A good insurance is to take a fiber supplement like psyllium husks.
Flavones	Flavones prevent testosterone from being transformed into estrogen.	Onions and green tea are the best sources of flavones.
Green tea	Green tea lowers levels of less healthy estrogen while black tea can raise them.	Green tea in all forms including a quality green tea supplement.
Antioxidants	Antioxidants help stimulate detoxifying enzymes and blocks estrogen receptors on cell membranes, reducing the risk of breast and cervical cancers.	Cruciferous veggies like broccoli, cabbage, kale, and Brussels sprouts. Adding green tea and supplements help to increase antioxidants.

Increase Estrogen With:	What Happens:	Sources:
Alcohol	Postmenopausal women who have 1 drink a day increase estrogen levels by 7%... 2 drinks a day increases estrogen by 22%.	If you're at any risk for breast cancer, your best bet is to skip the alcohol. If you do choose to drink, have a maximum of 1 drink a day.
Caffeine	300 mg of caffeine increases estrogen levels.	Limit yourself to 1 or 2 cups of coffee a day...and skip the soda, which does nothing good for our body. Green tea would be a helpful swap.
Trans Fat	Trans fats are bad all around! It increases belly fat, which stimulates estrogen production.	Most pre-packaged foods are filled with trans-fats. Always check the labels and be aware of false claims of "trans-fat free." Avoid fried or prepackaged foods that say partially hydrogenated oils on the ingredients list.
Yams	Yams decrease the metabolism of estrogen that leads to a buildup in our body. They are also high in carbohydrates.	Stick to ½ cup; to have a hormonal effect, we're talking about at least 2 yams a day.
Milk	Hormones given to cows to fatten them up can transfer into their milk supply, causing young girls to have their menstrual cycle at earlier ages.	We are the only species that drinks milk after infancy...hmmm interesting! Try to almond milk or coconut milk.

Increase Estrogen With:	What Happens:	Sources:
Flaxseeds	Flaxseed is a great fiber and omega 3 fat to include in your diet. It also contains a phytoestrogen-like compound that can support healthy estrogen levels and can help reduce hot flashes.	Buy whole flaxseeds, and grind up a little at a time (I use a coffee grinder). To keep omega 3's fresh, store in the refrigerator. Add ground flaxseeds to smoothies, or baked goods (I add it to my muffin recipes).
Using plastic	Never microwave in plastic! It leaches unhealthy estrogen into our cells.	Try not to use the microwave and don't drink from plastic water bottles.
Soy (fermented vs. concentrated forms)	Soy contains phytoestrogens called isoflavones; which mimics and increases estrogen. A jail was fined because they served their prisoners all soy to decrease their testosterone and increase estrogen…not a good combination for our health or metabolism!	Stay away from concentrated products, such as soy milk, soy nuts or soy nut-butter.

Testosterone

Most people think of testosterone as a male hormone, but it is something women also have and need for many functions in our body. How much our body produces depends on our gender, time of day, age, eating habits, sleep patterns, menstrual cycle, menopause, stress, and medications. In men, testosterone is produced in the testes. In women, ovaries and the adrenal glands produce testosterone. Unfortunately, optimal levels decline with age. Diet, exercise, medications can all affect the levels of testosterone.

Testosterone is essential for these 6 issues:

1. It preserves muscle mass
2. It facilitates sex drive
3. It regulates moods
4. It builds energy
5. It enhances nutrition
6. High levels form masculine traits

Testosterone enhances muscle development, decreases fat stores, and increases bone mass. It also plays an important role for determining our moods, depression, energy levels, ability to have orgasms, and ability to sleep; along with other hormones. Scientists discovered that the higher the testosterone levels, the higher the levels of good HDL cholesterol and the lower the levels of bad LDL cholesterol.

Low testosterone levels have been directly linked to many undesired health issues, including low sperm count, erectile dysfunction, low energy, mood changes and weak bones. Low testosterone levels can increase body fat, particularly abdominal fat, and deadly medical conditions such as type 2 diabetes and heart disease. If you have low testosterone levels, the body easily burns up muscle instead of the desired fuel of fat and carbohydrates; which is often shown by skinny legs and bulging stomachs.

So how do we hold onto our calorie-burning muscles? Muscles need protein. Hormones, like testosterone and human growth hormone, help proteins find their way to muscles and stay there. They also help preserve muscle once it has been made, and help the body burn fat instead. If it wasn't for these hormones, protein from food could not create new muscles, and existing muscles would get quickly burned up for energy.

Low testosterone levels can be caused by many factors, including being overweight. A study in 2006 followed testosterone levels of 2,100 men age 45 and older. They discovered that the obese men were 2.4 times more likely to have low testosterone compared to men at a healthy weight. Studies have also found that as Body Mass Index (BMI) increases, there is a direct connection to a decline of testosterone levels.

Weight loss in general can enhance testosterone. Researchers measured testosterone levels in two groups of middle-aged obese men. One group followed a 4 month weight-loss program while a second group did nothing. The weight-loss group lost an average of 45 pounds and also had notable increases in testosterone levels. More and more studies are linking body weight and testosterone levels. The human body has an intricate system of hormones that interact in a multitude of complex ways. The relationship between testosterone and weight is part of a large sequence of physiological processes that can be improved through diet and exercise.

We can't do anything about the natural progression of our biological clocks, but we can take control over our weight. Since testosterone production is known to decrease in direct proportion to the level of obesity, it is crucial to maintain a healthy weight; and not just for testosterone, but for every aspect of our health.

BALANCE YOUR TESTOSTERONE LEVELS

Too little testosterone can lead to muscle loss, dry skin and poor elasticity, a decreased libido and bone density loss. Most people want to increase their levels of testosterone. However, if you are a woman suffering from Polycystic Ovarian Syndrome keeping your testosterone levels on the down-low is important. The signs of too much testosterone include increased abdominal fat, acne, irregular periods, hair loss, irritability, and a decrease in breast size.

Increase Testosterone With:	What happens	Sources
Fat	An increase in the amount of fat in your diet increases the amount of testosterone.	Eat quality fats like butter, avocados, nuts, and coconut oil. Organic meat and dairy products (never consume fat-free versions) are great sources of protein and fat.

Increase Testosterone With:	What happens	Sources
Allicin	A study found that allicin added to a high-protein diet increased testosterone levels. It also decreases cortisol, which competes with testosterone and interferes with its normal function.	Add garlic and onions to your meals to stimulate testosterone's production.
Protein	Eating protein after intense exercise has been shown to increase the amount of testosterone that enters muscle cells which stimulates muscle growth.	Choose quality protein, and try supplementing whey protein (especially after exercise). Or use whey in baked goods to sneak in a protein boost!
Cruciferous veggies	Cabbage, broccoli, cauliflower and other cruciferous veggies contain nutrients called indoles. Indoles lower estrogen which also competes with testosterone production.	Increase your consumption of raw broccoli, Brussels sprouts, cauliflower and cabbage.
B Vitamins	Studies show that consumption of B Vitamins directly correlates with an increase in testosterone.	Meat, poultry, and fish contain lots of b vitamins. Vegetarians should be sure to take a b-complex vitamin.
Caffeine	High amounts of caffeine added to exercise can increase testosterone production.	Don't go crazy with this fact. Stick to 200-400mg of caffeine a day and keep caffeine away from bed-time. Sleep is just as important to testosterone.
Niacin	Studies show that niacin increases HDL; which directly links to a higher testosterone production.	Increase niacin by including meat, poultry, fish, nuts, eggs and quality dairy products.

Increase Testosterone With:	What happens	Sources
Zinc	A deficiency in zinc can cause a 75% drop in testosterone. Zinc supplements can cause testosterone levels to double if deficient and can increase sperm production in men.	Zinc is found in most protein sources. Oysters and seafood are great sources. Beef, pork, dark meat poultry, Cheddar cheese, and almonds also have high levels of zinc.
Stinging nettle	Supplement with stinging nettle root extract, as this has been shown to help free testosterone from sex hormone-binding globulin (SHBG).	Supplement your diet with stinging nettle; which can be found at your local health food store.
Exercise	After about 20 minutes into an exercise session, blood levels of testosterone increase and remain elevated for up to three hours after exercise.	Maintain muscle with consistent strength training.

Reduce Testosterone With:	What Happens	Sources
Alcohol	Drinking alcohol increases estrogen; which in turn decreases testosterone.	Stay away from alcohol. If needed keep drinks to a minimum.
Low-fat diet	A low-fat diet nullifies the typical increase in testosterone after resistance training.	Include a balance of fat and protein after a tough workout. I love coconut oil for this!

Reduce Testosterone With:	What Happens	Sources
Low-protein diet	Low-protein diets increase sex hormone-binding globulin (SHBG) levels; which attaches to hormones and makes them unavailable for our body. An increase in SHBG decreases usable testosterone.	Always include a protein at every meal and snack.
Phytoestrogens	Phytoestrogens mimic estrogen; which in turn decreases testosterone.	Phytoestrogens are found in flaxseeds and soy products; keep these to a minimum.
Lack of sleep and too much stress	Getting less than 7 hours of sleep a night decreases the production of testosterone. An increase in stress boosts the secretion of cortisol; which overshadows the production of testosterone.	Get sufficient sleep and reduce stress.

DHEA

Scientists who study obesity recognize losing excess weight is difficult. Indeed, as many as 95% of dieters gain back unwanted weight, getting caught in end-less cycles of yo-yo dieting. Researchers have concluded the human body has a genetically determined set-point weight that's controlled by metabolic hormones. One of these essential metabolic hormones is DHEA. DHEA is a steroid hormone that is produced by the adrenal glands; its full name is Dehydroepiandrosterone. The body converts DHEA to male and female sex hormones, such as estrogen and testosterone.

As we age, our body's production of DHEA decreases. Many scientists are now calling this hormone the "fountain of youth." DHEA levels peak at about age 20 and by age 40 we produce half the DHEA that we did at age 20; by 65, our bodies are producing about 15% of the DHEA we produced at age 20. This decline has been linked to many common negative effects of aging as well as many degenerative conditions such as cancer, hardening of the arteries, a slowed immune system, loss of memory and a general lack of energy; which is why there has been substantial attention to DHEA and its role in aging. In fact, DHEA supplements have been referred to as an anti-aging hormone because people with lower levels of DHEA have been reported to suffer from adrenal deficiency, kidney disease, type 2 diabetes, breast cancer, heart disease, and osteoporosis. Certain medications may also deplete DHEA, such as corticosteroids, insulin, opiates and danazol.

Our body has specific DHEA receptors, proving that DHEA directly affects our body. DHEA is also in charge of stimulating hormones that control fat metabolism as well as stress. In general, it is responsible for preserving our youthful vitality, a lean body and many other desirable traits of youth.

Therefore, it seems likely that it would be of great benefit to find a way to compensate for the decline of DHEA levels as we age. By eating properly we may find a way to possibly reverse the aging process, creating a "fountain of youth."

One of the most exciting benefits of DHEA is its ability to burn fat and helps keep it off by converting fat to muscle; instead of storing calories as fat, DHEA assists by burning calories for energy. Some scientists claim that this discovery may be one of the "most significant finds in weight control of this century," because no matter what you eat, weight loss still occurs.

DHEA appears to create a stabilizing effect on all body systems. Instead of weight loss due to the breakdown of lean muscle tissue or fluid loss, DHEA is claimed to directly help the body build lean muscle tissue. Apparently DHEA blocks G6PD (glucose-6-phosphate-dehyrogenase), the main enzyme in charge of the production of fat tissue as well as cancer cells. By blocking G6PD, it helps to stop the production of these two unfavorable conditions.

Studies have found that people with higher DHEA levels tend to live longer, healthier lives than those with lower levels. The Food and Drug Administration removed DHEA supplements from the market in 1985 due to false claims about health benefits. The US Dietary Supplement Health and Education Act of 1994 revived DHEA supplements to the market and its popularity continues to grow. Despite this growth and attention, support for the health claims, particularly as tested on people, is lacking. Therefore, I bring your awareness to nutrition and how that can help increase and maintain your DHEA levels.

BALANCE YOUR DHEA LEVELS

Keeping our DHEA levels high is essential to our youthful vigor. Referred to as our "fountain of youth," I definitely want to keep this hormone pumping strong! DHEA that is raised naturally within the body is the safest.

Increase DHEA with:	What Happens:	Sources:
Exercise	DHEA can be naturally increased in the body with exercise.	Any type of exercise will help, but strength training really gets DHEA going!
Fat and Omega 3's	Omega-3's can play a big part in raising your DHEA. The more calories from fat in a diet, the higher their DHEA levels.	Eat plenty of foods with omega-3 fatty acids such as those found in salmon and CLAs from grass-fed meat.
Chromium	Chromium picolinate increases DHEA levels.	Broccoli is a good source of chromium.
Magnesium	Most people suffer from a magnesium deficiency. An adequate amount of magnesium increases secretion of DHEA.	Leafy green vegetables, nuts and seeds are good sources of magnesium. A magnesium glycinate supplement just before bed is extremely beneficial (see supplement chapter).

Increase DHEA with:	What Happens:	Sources:
Vitamin E	Studies found that taking vitamin E can boost DHEA. In turn, DHEA prevents breakdown of vitamin E in the body.	Nuts and green leafy vegetables are good food sources of vitamin E.
Plant phytosterols	The nutrients found in plant phytosterols can naturally increase production of DHEA.	Found in vegetables, nuts, seeds and other plant sources.
Sleep	When you don't get adequate sleep, your adrenal glands get depleted and can't produce the required amount of DHEA.	Get around 8 hours of sleep; not just for DHEA secretion, but for a healthy balance in every hormone in our body!

Decrease DHEA with:	What Happens:	Solutions
Too many carbohydrates	Carbohydrates decrease DHEA levels in the body. A diet high in carbohydrates not only decreases DHEA, but it can also hold back weight loss.	Stick to quality carbohydrates with plenty of fiber; such as non-starchy vegetables. Stay away from refined carbohydrates.
Low-fat, high-fiber diet	Too much fiber can decrease DHEA levels, but studies find that when you resume a high-fat diet, DHEA levels go back up. Fiber may reduce re-absorption of DHEA once it has been moved through the liver.	Fiber is helpful in so many ways, so rather than decreasing fiber intake, increase healthy fats in your diet. Focus on omega'3s and CLAs from coconut oil, grass-fed beef, and organic butter.
Caffeine	Caffeine can lower DHEA levels and raise cortisol levels, increasing stress and anxiety.	Stick to 200mg a day if needed, or switch to decaf.

Decrease DHEA with:	What Happens:	Solutions
Alcohol	Alcohol decreases DHEA serum levels.	Stick to one glass of red wine a day if needed, but even better…stay away from alcohol to enhance the balance of all our hormones.
Soy Isoflavones	Concentrated amounts of soy Isoflavones can decrease your DHEA levels by 32%.	Stay away from concentrated soy isoflavones like soy milk and soy butter.
Stress	Stress can suppress DHEA levels in the body.	Try to reduce as much stress in your life as possible. Meditation or yoga can be a great way to relieve stress.

Cortisol

Whenever we're anxious, angry, scared, or tense, our brain stimulates the production of cortisol and adrenaline; which are hormones distinctively designed to rouse the fight-or-flight response that was once essential to our survival. Adrenaline's role is to make you aware and focused. Cortisol increases heart rate and tenses your muscles to get them ready for the stressors ahead.

While those physiological developments were important for our prehistoric ancestors, they're not so helpful in a world where physical dangers are few. Whenever we're stressed these hormones are stimulated into our system. Once the stress has decreased, adrenaline levels fall, but cortisol remains high. Since your body thinks you've run a mile or done something physical in response to the 'threat', cortisol sends signals to refuel the body as soon as possible. It's an uncontrollable feeling to treat yourself with foods loaded in carbohydrates that leads to weight gain and health issues to those who are chronically stressed. It can cause a blood sugar imbalance and can cause you to eat more than you need. It's a nasty cycle of stress…increased cortisol… cookie, cake, ice cream…weight gain!

The type of weight gain this cycle increases is also discouraging. Cortisol and adrenaline travel to fat cells, signaling them to open and release fat into the bloodstream, to the liver and then to the muscles to use as energy. The scary problem is that fat cells deep inside the belly are particularly good at attracting cortisol. The cycle of hormonal responses caused by stress promotes the buildup of excess 'stress fat' in the layer of fat below the abdominal muscle. Belly fat is the worse type of fat; this creates "toxic weight" which is the type of fat linked to heart disease, high blood pressure, stroke, cancer and diabetes.

Although we can't eliminate external stress from our lives, there are some steps we can take. Controlling cortisol levels with diet and exercise can stop that unpleasant belly fat from accumulating. Watch out for certain foods that can stimulate more stress and concentrate on relaxing exercise; such as yoga, which is very therapeutic for decreasing cortisol.

BALANCE YOUR CORTISOL LEVELS

Unfortunately, in today's world, we all experience significant amounts of stress, and it doesn't appear to be going away anytime soon. Our daily lives naturally increase cortisol levels. Things we do and put in our mouths everyday can help keep this fat-storing hormone low. For some of us, our relationship with food is just another addition to stress levels. Here are some foods and solutions to help decrease stress when times get tough.

Decrease Cortisol with:	What Happens:	Sources:
Whey Protein	The amino acid, tryptophan, in whey protein boosts serotonin and decreases cortisol.	Try adding whey protein powder to breakfast shakes and baked goods; cortisol is highest in the morning!
Omega 3's	High levels of omega-3 will help get rid of this deadly visceral fat because the essential fatty acids decrease cortisol levels.	Choose foods like wild Alaskan salmon, anchovies, sardines, and other cold-water fish, along with fish oil capsules.

Decrease Cortisol with:	What Happens:	Sources.
B-Vitamins	B vitamins help develop and maintain the nervous system which is in overdrive during times of stress. They also help convert calories from food into energy in the body.	Include turkey, liver, tuna, chili peppers, and tempeh (soy). Other meats, dairy products and eggs are high in vitamin B12. Brewer's yeast, avocado, salmon, Brazil nuts are also good sources.
High-fiber foods	Fiber lowers cortisol. Carbohydrates filled with fiber don't cause an insulin spike so cortisol levels don't spike either.	Focus on a balance of both types of fiber; soluble and insoluble.
Green Tea	Theanine is a unique amino acid found in the leaves of green tea and acts as a stress reliever. Theanine in green tea may be effective in combating tension, stress, and anxiety without inducing drowsiness.	Green tea in all forms. A supplement can also be helpful.
Beta-sitosterol	Beta-sitosterol regulates the stress response by managing cortisol levels within a normal range. Beta-sitosterol has been also shown to rebuild desired hormones such as DHEA.	Plant oils contain the highest concentration of beta-sitosterol; veggies, nuts and seeds contain fairly high levels.
Antioxidants	Studies found that antioxidants prevent other physical signs of stress. Cortisol levels were 3 times higher in participants that did not receive antioxidants. Antioxidants are released from the adrenals during stress; adding these could help support this significant gland.	All vegetables contain some amount of antioxidants. Add in green peppers, tomatoes, broccoli, and other leafy greens to your diet.

Decrease Cortisol with:	What Happens:	Sources:
Glutamine	High cortisol levels break down muscle proteins resulting in the release of glutamine into the blood. Research has shown that glutamine counteracts the effects of cortisol and maintains muscle under stressful conditions.	Doctors suggest supplementation in a range from 5 to 40 grams per day. Athletes may need higher doses to notice an effect (see supplement chapter).

Increase Cortisol with:	What Happens:	Sources:
Alcohol	Alcohol activates the hypothalamic-pituitary-adrenal axis, causing the adrenals to produce more cortisol.	Studies show that heavy drinking brings up cortisol levels. One study did find that a glass of white wine actually lowers cortisol. Bottom line: Stick to one or less drinks a day.
Sugar	Cortisol lowers serotonin levels, encouraging us to crave sugar and eat more of it. Weight gain can result from this altered chemistry. The more sugar we eat, the more our blood sugar levels plummet, causing us to feel even worse.	Limit your sugar as much as possible and check ingredient lists; sugar is hidden in ketchup, marinara sauce, salad dressings...
Caffeine	Caffeine increases cortisol by elevating secretion of adrenocorticotrophic; which is cortisol's precursor hormone.	Stick to one cup a day or switch to decaf. Green tea would be a very helpful change.
Capsaicin and hot peppers	This hot food causes adrenal glands to release epinephrine, norepinephrine, and cortisol, but only for a short time. An hour after this brief rise your adrenal hormones may fall even lower than before the ingestion of capsaicin.	Capsaicin can also reduce inflammation, pain, heart disease, cancer, and ulcers, so Capsaicin has many benefits too.

Increase Cortisol with:	What Happens:	Sources:
Gluten	Gluten is the protein in wheat products, which turns to a "glue" in our intestines. Gluten intolerance increases cortisol levels. Many people are sensitive to gluten and don't realize it. Try to eliminate gluten to see if you feel better.	Stay away from wheat, rye and barley. There are tons of "gluten free" products out there. Check out my chapter on "Alternative Flours."
Licorice	Glycyrrhetinic acid in licorice stops an enzyme that inactivates cortisol. Eating licorice extends the life of cortisol in the kidneys.	Stay away from licorice candy; Twizzlers are made almost entirely out of high fructose corn syrup.
Refined carbs	Carbohydrates increase insulin, another hormone that plays an important role in weight gain and appetite. Elevated cortisol and insulin levels are a 'lethal duo' that creates an insatiable appetite for carbohydrates.	Avoiding foods that release sugar into the bloodstream too quickly. Watch out for highly processed foods made with white, refined sugars and white starches; such as pasta, white rice, potatoes, white bread, and foods with added sugars.
Inadequate Sleep	A sleep-deprived night creates a consistently elevated level of cortisol, which encourages your cells to store more fat, particularly when paired with insulin resistance.	Always aim for 8 hours of sleep a night.
Very restrictive diet with over-exercise	High intensity exercise and/or a very restricted calorie intake can produce additional physical stress on the body that may trigger even more cortisol production. The higher the cortisol levels, the greater the tendency to gain fat in the middle of the body.	Take a moderate approach with both diet and exercise. Moderate low intensity aerobic exercise is most suitable for people in this situation as it helps burn calories without significantly increasing cortisol levels.

CHAPTER 7

SLEEP

Sleep and Weight loss

Do you often plan on losing weight in the summer but end up gaining? One reason for this phenomenon is the longer days and less sleep! My clients love when I give them the assignment of getting more sleep. Some lose 4 pounds without changing their diet and adding a few hours of sleep a night. One of my heavier clients lost 17 pounds in 6 days just by adding natural sleep supplements. This helped her increase her sleep from 2 hours a night to 7. According to the National Sleep Foundation, most people need at least eight hours of high-quality sleep every night. I say "high-quality" because a night brought on by Tylenol PM or alcohol is not quality sleep. Quality sleep is when our bodies get into the rapid eye movement state. REM or rapid eye movement sleep is a peak time for growth and repair and if we don't get enough, our health and metabolism will suffer.

Sleep deprivation impairs our ability to metabolize carbohydrates and increases our stress hormones. This can lead to high blood sugar, high insulin levels and weight gain. If you are staying awake to get more things done, surf the internet, or watch TV you are not alone. Our society seems to reward people for working more and sleeping less. The pharmaceutical industry encourages this dysfunctional sleep pattern by offering drugs to help you fall asleep and drugs to help you wake up. Now is the time for us to start making an effort to get more sleep. Chronic sleep deprivation can have a variety of effects on the metabolism and overall health. Here are some problems that follow sleep deprivation:

- It interfere with the body's ability to metabolize carbohydrates and causes high blood levels of glucose, which leads to higher insulin levels and insulin is our "fat-storing" hormone.
- It decreases leptin production, which causes an intense desire for carbohydrates.
- Reduces human growth hormone production, which is our 'fat-burning' hormone
- Causes imbalances in our neurotransmitters and increases depression and anxiety
- Increased risk of diabetes
- Increases blood pressure
- Increased risk of heart disease
- Increases obesity
- Increase rates of breast cancer
- Increase memory loss

LACK OF SLEEP AND HORMONES

Many studies connect a link between sleep and the hormones that manipulate our eating behavior; which are ghrelin and leptin. Have you ever experienced a sleepless night followed by a day when no matter what you ate you never felt satisfied? This is the outcome when leptin and ghrelin get out of balance. Leptin and ghrelin work like a "checks and balances" that manage hunger and fullness. Ghrelin, produced in the stomach, increases appetite, while leptin, produced in fat cells, sends a message to our brain when we are full. A lack of sleep causes ghrelin levels to increase and your leptin levels to decrease. This imbalance causes us to intensely crave food and never feel full. The worst part is that we don't crave broccoli…we crave high calorie sweets and starchy foods. Over time, this imbalance can easily lead to long-term weight gain.

In a Chicago study, doctors analyzed leptin and ghrelin levels in 12 fit men. They started by charting their normal levels of appetite and hunger. The men were assigned to two days of sleep deprivation followed by two days of limitless sleep. Doctors supervised hormone levels, appetite, and activity level. The men had considerable changes. When sleep was restricted, leptin levels went down and ghrelin levels went up. As expected, the men's appetite also increased; **the desire for high carbohydrate, high calorie foods increased by a shocking 45 percent.**

A Stanford study found an interesting significance of the leptin-ghrelin effect. They studied 1,000 volunteers that reported the number of hours they slept each night. Doctors then analyzed their levels of ghrelin and leptin, and their weight. The numbers show that the volunteers who slept less than eight hours a night not only had lower levels of leptin and higher levels of ghrelin, but they also had a higher body fat levels. The link comes when they discovered that their levels of body fat correlated with their sleep patterns. Those who slept the fewest hours per night weighed the most.

Don't throw your walking shoes away just because this is an easier way to lose weight. Studies also show the relationship is not as obvious as it seems. An interesting problem called, "obstructive sleep apnea," is something that most people have without knowing it. This causes an imbalance in our hormone levels. People with sleep apnea stop breathing for up to a minute, sometimes hundreds of times throughout the night. It is mysterious because the true cause of the problem is unknown. Some doctors believe that a physical deformity inside the throat cause soft tissue to collapse. This briefly pinches the air passages during a night, causing a disruption in breathing and a tendency to snore. So even though you are unconscious for eight hours, the disrupted breathing stops you from getting quality sleep. Eight hours of disrupted sleep can leave you feeling like you had only a 4 or 5. One symptom of sleep apnea is that you wake up feeling tired even though you thought you went to bed early. People who suffer from sleep apnea are more likely to be overweight. The confusing part is that doctors find they have oddly high levels of leptin; which turns off hunger. Another interesting fact is that when their apnea is treated, leptin levels drop and somehow that helps them to lose weight. Confused? Me too...

As it turns out, the level of this hormone doesn't matter as much as our response to it. I began to understand when they compared this to people who are "insulin resistant," they have plenty of insulin but their body can't recognize it because they became de-sensitized. People with apnea are resistant to the fullness signal that leptin sends to the brain. The body is trying to tell them to stop eating, but the brain isn't getting the message. Experts believe our exercise patterns, eating habits, stress levels, and genetics all control the production and response of leptin and ghrelin.

Sleeping less also affects changes in our basal metabolic rate (remember from chapter one: the number of calories you burn when you rest). When you are sleeping, your body produces human growth hormone; the stuff celebrities are now injecting to look young and feel young. Human growth hormone helps preserve our muscle and keep our metabolism firing at night. So an inadequate amount of sleep will keep this highly desired hormone from kicking in. Another thing to remember is that our human growth hormone doesn't kick in if we eat 3 hours before bed.

The book, "The Thyroid Diet: Manage Your Metabolism for Lasting Weight Loss," explains the impact of sleep on cortisol levels. A lack of sleep increases the release of the stress hormone, cortisol, and stimulates hunger and tells us to hold onto those carbohydrates in our belly fat. A lack of sleep can also slow our thyroid hormones; which has a huge impact on our metabolism.

Another piece to the weight connection that is called non-exercise associated thermogenesis; which is unplanned activity, such as fidgeting (chapter one). If you sleep less, you move around less, and burn up fewer calories.

When you get a good night's rest your body has adequate time to repair and rejuvenate. Adults need between 7 and 9 hours of quality sleep a night for optimal health. Children and teenagers require even more. Some people just don't have enough time in the day to get enough sleep, but millions of Americans chronically experience trouble falling asleep, waking in the night or both. Here are some tips I use to help me get 8 hours of quality sleep.

- Avoid sugar and foods high in carbohydrates, like popcorn, chips, and crackers, in the evening hours. It causes low quality sleep because when blood sugar rises, it must fall which will cause us to wake up in the middle of the night.
- Follow a regular sleep schedule by going to bed and rising at the same time.
- Before bed do something to relax your muscles and your mind (stretching, yoga or deep breathing exercises).

- Reduce or eliminate caffeine...chocolate has caffeine, so beware.
- Turn off the T.V. and computer and darken your bedroom with heavy drapes.
- Turn the heat down. I often sleep with the windows open even in the winter; I sleep the best at about 57 degrees.
- Add in natural supplements.

If these healthy habits don't solve your insomnia, I and millions of Americans use 400 to 800 mg of Magnesium Glycinate at bedtime. This mineral is a natural muscle relaxant and can help calm anxiety, both of which help with sleep. "The Magnesium Miracle" is an amazing book that explains in detail. If this does not work, then it is time to contact a health professional or nutritionist to inquire about progesterone cream, 5-HTP or melatonin. These are effective and natural ways to improve sleep. We are all pressed for time but I encourage you to find eight hours for sleep to maximize energy, mood, mental focus and metabolism. It is the easiest way to maximize our health, no painful exercises required.

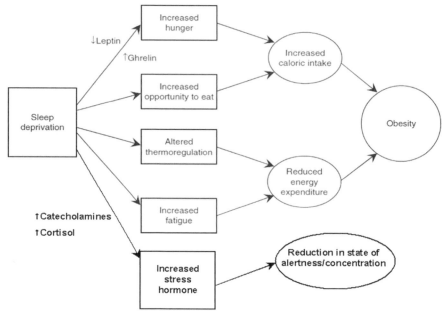

Graph from: "Short Sleep Duration and Weight Gain: A Systematic Review" - Sanjay R. Patel and Frank B. Hu, 2007

CHAPTER 8

ENHANCING OUR HEALTH WITH SUPPLEMENTS

Weight loss and cellular energy

A large piece of the weight loss puzzle is cellular energy production. Many diet products contain stimulants which unnaturally stimulate thermogenesis also known as the production of energy and heat; such as ephedra. These may work for a while, but they leave you feeling tired and edgy when they wear off. Resveratrol, green tea, l-carnitine, coenzyme Q10, CLA and alpha-lipoic acid are some nutrients that are found in food which in therapeutic doses naturally optimize your body's cellular energy production. Not only do these nutrients provide greater energy and endurance, and a greater ability to lose body fat, they help prevent aging in our cells. The food you eat and your exercise regime will work in combination with your cellular energy production to either lead to weight loss or gain.

Many of you may ask...are these safe to take? Yet you won't think twice about popping an Advil because commercials claim it will take care of your "aches and pains." Advil is a chemical that is foreign to our body, where the supplements I believe in are either found in food (only in concentrated- therapeutic doses) or found in our body (we just need more of it, like Co-enzyme Q10). Here are some top supplements to aid in a healthy and strong metabolism.

The benefits of exercise are widely known and understood, but unfortunately, the potential negative effects have only recently been addressed in the athletic community. Could exercise actually be causing damage to your body? It's ironic, but it's true. Exercise causes elevated aerobic metabolism, which in turn increases the production of killer molecules known as free radicals.

A free radical is a molecule that's missing at least one electron in its outermost orbit, which causes it to be negatively charged. Like most things in nature, free radicals seek to remain neutral, and in an effort to achieve this balance they bump up against healthy cells in your body and steal electrons from them. This process is similar to an electric shock that leaves the once healthy cell, damaged and mutated.

Unfortunately the process doesn't stop after damaging the first cell. This newly damaged molecule is now also missing an electron and becomes a free radical. Each free radical that is created zaps electrons from healthy molecules to form new free radicals which generate a chain reaction that damages thousands of cells along its path.

Scared? I hope so, because scientists now believe that free radical damage increases cellular deterioration, which is associated with accelerated aging, cancer, diabetes and coronary artery disease. This is ironic because the human body is designed to regenerate most of its cells. Our bones, skin and blood cells all regenerate over time to slow the aging process. Free radicals, however, replace cellular regeneration with cellular degeneration, which ultimately speeds up the aging process.

Free radical damage has become more prevalent in our society as witnessed by the increase in cancer victims in recent years. Environmental pollutants like smog, cigarette smoke and car exhaust all contain free radical molecules, and as our exposure to these increase, so does our chances of degenerative diseases. Worse yet, research illustrate that mental stress is one of the highest causes of free radicals.

The good news is that under normal conditions your body has the natural ability to defend against free radicals by producing three substances; glutathione, catalase and superoxide dismutase. These substances are known as antioxidants, which work as free radical scavengers by seeking them out and donating the electrons needed to neutralize them, thereby quenching their need to search out and destroy healthy cells. Antioxidants reduce muscle fatigue and post-exercise muscle soreness. They also have an alkalinizing effect on the body, making it less acidic, which promotes muscle mass maintenance.

The problem occurs when free radical production exceeds the body's ability to produce antioxidants. This can happen during intense exercise when athletes use 10 to 20 times the amount of oxygen than that of a sedentary person. During exercise, the conversion of fat and sugar into energy occurs through a process known as oxidation. During this process, most of the oxygen combines with hydrogen to produce water. However, about 5% of the oxygen forms free radicals.

Imagine that, every time you breathe, free radicals are formed. This process of oxidation is similar to what you see when metal rusts or an apple slice turns brown from exposure to air. Your body can defend against normal levels of free radicals, but if you exercise, live in a polluted area, or have a stressful life, as most of us do, then supplementing your diet with antioxidants may be of great value.

A well balanced diet with plenty of vegetables is important and will help, but alone it's just not enough. Factory processing, additives and pesticides all work to destroy antioxidants within our foods and nutrient depleted soils no longer provide us with the nutrient rich foods that our grandparents enjoyed.

Eating a well-balanced diet and a taking strong Multi-Vitamin/Mineral/Antioxidant Supplement each day should be considered for adequate antioxidant protection and to promote optimum performance and long-term health. There's a saying, "Take care of your body for the first 50 years of your life, and it will take care of you for next 50." Antioxidant protection and good diet is a great way to start.

Most athletes need more vitamins and minerals than sedentary people and vitamin deficiencies can create difficulties in training and recovery. Most of the data suggests that increased intake of vitamin E is protective against exercise induced oxidative damage. It is hypothesized that vitamin E is also involved in the recovery process following exercise.

You have the capability of lessening the harm caused from free radical destruction on muscle tissue and the immune system. It means better recovery from your intense workouts, which results in more frequent exercise sessions by decreasing time needed to facilitate muscular repair and cardiovascular conditioning. It also means you're less likely to become ill from the flu or cold, which can sideline your progress.

With antioxidant support, your immune system is more resilient and you have more energy because you free up otherwise burdened cellular activity, therefore increasing your metabolism, enabling energy producing cellular processes. The cellular membranes are better protected, and are better able to hold on to nutrients, water, proteins, and glycogen stores vital for growth, repair and energy. I believe antioxidants to be more important to the athletic person than any ergogenic (energy-generating) sports supplement on the market today!

The main antioxidant in the human body is glutathione. Glutathione is a tri-peptide amino acid formed from glutamic acid, cysteine, and glycine. Glutathione is produced in the liver and is a major defender against this free radical attack. It detoxifies harmful compounds, aids immune function, strengthens red and white blood cell count, and functions as a neurotransmitter. Glutathione also protects cell membranes including the mitochondria (fat-burning furnace) from harmful oxidative stress. Glutathione also protects the surface of the cell membrane and supports other antioxidants that in turn help glutathione. For example; one intense bout of exercise to exhaustion can reduce muscle glutathione levels by 40% and liver glutathione by 80% and continues to decline thereafter. You cannot prevent muscle damage and maintain training intensity without sufficient supplies of this vital component.

There are several antioxidants that have a positive effect on the amount of glutathione in our liver and cells. Some work by directly increasing glutathione production and others protect glutathione activity. The following antioxidants help to defend against free radical formation, with some supporting glutathione production as well.

Vitamin C: Ascorbic acid is a water soluble vitamin present in citrus fruits, green peppers, cabbage, spinach, broccoli, kale, cantaloupe, and strawberries. The RDA is 60 mg per day. Intake above 2000 mg may be associated with adverse side effects in some individuals. Aids in the formation of collagen (glue that holds the body together), hormone and neurotransmitter synthesis, enhances immune function including assisting white blood cell activity. Promotes healing, and aids in recovery from illness and physical exertion.

Vitamin E: A fat soluble vitamin present in nuts, coconut flour, seeds, vegetable and fish oils, eggs and Just Like Sugar (see alternative sweeteners). Current recommended daily allowance (RDA) is 15 IU per day for men and 12 IU per day for women. It actually hides in the cell membrane waiting for free radicals in which to neutralize. It improves circulation, prevents and repairs tissue cells, and helps protect other fat-soluble antioxidants. Like vitamin C, it has been proven effective in many degenerative illness and conditions.

Beta-carotene is a precursor to vitamin A, or retinol, and is present in liver, egg yolk, cream, butter, spinach, broccoli, and tomato. Because beta-carotene is converted to vitamin A by the body there is no set requirement. Instead the RDA is expressed as retinol equivalents (RE), to clarify the relationship. They enhance immune function and maintain and repair cellular processes. It is important to note that vitamin A has no antioxidant properties and can be quite toxic when taken in excess.

Melatonin: Besides aiding in good quality sleep, this hormone, produced by the pineal gland, enhances immune function, protects against cancer, aids in stress reduction, and boosts glutathione production. Due to its size, melatonin has the ability to saturate just about every cell in the human body. It's also one of the most powerful naturally occurring antioxidants ever found. It has been shown effective against many of the age related and chronic degenerative conditions known today. It seems to influence just about every immune enhancing and antioxidant producing system in the human body. It is found in very small amounts in food.

The following are other potent antioxidants that have a place in the cellular anti-oxidative protocol:

✓ Coenzyme Q10
✓ Resveratrol
✓ Garlic
✓ Alpha-Lipolic Acid
✓ Acetyl-L-Carnitine
✓ Green Tea
✓ Manganese

The body has built-in defense mechanisms to repair itself. But with the stresses of today, exercise, sickness and an inferior diet, free radical damage may get out of hand. Just look at all the diseases and health conditions today. It is my suggestion that, at the very least, you should take a multi-vitamin/mineral supplement. The athlete and anyone else environmentally, physically, or mentally challenged should consider not only a good multi-vitamin/mineral supplement, but also should consider supplementing antioxidants.

Supplement #2 Green tea

Green tea is an antioxidant-rich beverage; which can also be concentrated in a supplement form. Green tea offers a wide array of health benefits including improved blood sugar, fat loss, improved circulation and cancer prevention.

Animal studies have found that supplementation with green tea extracts improves exercise endurance by increasing the muscles' fat-burning capacity. And in a 2008 human study from the University of Birmingham, England, acute supplementation with green tea extract increased fat burning during moderate-intensity exercise by 17 percent.

On a green tea weight loss diet study, sixty obese middle-aged women were placed on a diet of 1,800 calories per day. One group took a green tea supplement with breakfast, lunch, and dinner; the others took placebo pills. After two weeks on the green tea weight loss study, the women taking the diet pill had lost twice as much weight as the placebo group. After one month, the green tea group had three times the weight loss of the women who were only dieting.

Green tea increases the body's basal metabolic rate. This increase is referred to as a thermogenic effect; it assists with a weight loss program by helping the body burn more calories during day-to-day life. Tons of Japanese studies have been done that prove green tea contains thermogenic, calorie burning properties; which help us push through a weight loss plateau.

Green tea is also full of powerful antioxidants; so while your body burns fat faster, you are also providing your body with free radical killing polyphenols and flavanoids. The secret of green tea lies in the fact that it is rich in catechin polyphenols, particularly epigallocatechin gallate (EGCG). EGCG is a powerful antioxidant; which inhibits the growth of and kills cancer cells without harming healthy tissue. It has also been effective in lowering LDL cholesterol levels, and inhibiting the formation of blood clots.

Ancient China has used green tea for a variety of uses; it was used mainly against headaches and depression. Green tea has been shown in medical studies to fight against a wide array of health issues.
Increase fat oxidation and metabolism.
Reduces the level of cholesterol in blood, improves the ratio of good cholesterol to bad cholesterol.
Treat multiple sclerosis
Treatment and prevention of cancer
Reduce risk of Alzheimer's and Parkinson's diseases
Reduces the risk of heart diseases and heart attacks by reducing the risk of thrombosis
Reduces the risk of esophageal cancer
Inhibits the growth of certain cancer cells
Treat rheumatoid arthritis and cardiovascular diseases
Increases impaired immune function
Prevents tooth decay by killing the bacteria which causes the dental plaque

To date, the only negative side effect reported from drinking green tea is insomnia due to the fact that it contains caffeine. However, green tea contains less caffeine than coffee; it has about 30 milligrams of caffeine in eight ounces, compared to over one-hundred milligrams in eight ounces of coffee. If you have caffeine sensitivity please consult with your physician before embarking on the green tea journey.

The weight loss potential of green tea should be combined with a healthy diet and proper exercise. Drinking tons of cups of green tea can't hurt, but it isn't going to replace a sedentary lifestyle with a side of French fries.

Supplement #3 Resveratrol

Resveratrol is found in the skin of grapes and enhances our cardiovascular fitness, as well as brain, cellular and mental health. Until recently, this awesome antioxidant has been only found in red wine and in only insignificant amounts. Unless you drank a gallon of wine a day, you wouldn't consume enough resveratrol to see a difference, but now it is found in concentrated supplement forms.

Resveratrol speeds up your metabolism, burning off more calories and it also appears that it can be an appetite suppresser. Resveratrol isn't going to suck all your fat away while you continue to consume Oreos, but in addition to changing your eating habits for the long term (not just a month-long program), adding exercise with resveratrol will increase your success in your weight loss adventure.

Research proves that adding resveratrol increases metabolic activity, which can go a long way to not only losing weight, but maintaining a healthy weight. Resveratrol stimulates a gene called SIRT1, which is an anti-aging gene as well as a powerful fat burner. When SIRT1 is activated, weight gain is stalled by inhibiting fat storage. This awesome gene also slows the aging process because when the body is storing fewer fat cells, the undesired side effects that go along with aging, such as wrinkles and heart disease are also delayed.

Since resveratrol is an antioxidant, it also helps prevent free radical damage over the human body and offer better support to the blood vessels caused predominantly by high levels of blood glucose. Elevated levels of glucose in the blood can cause cellular damage; which increases problems with retinopathy, blindness, cancer, kidney and heart disease. A recent study found that resveratrol decreases age-related illnesses like Alzheimer's. Resveratrol also decreases arthritis, autoimmune diseases, and the risk of blood clotting.

The best way to take resveratrol is in the form of a multi supplement, combining it with other antioxidants to boost its powers. Most people combine green tea extract with resveratrol, which is also proven to enhance weight loss and is a potent antioxidant.

Doctors and scientists are true believers that resveratrol can decrease diabetes and insulin resistance in many people; two well-known problems of obesity. Resveratrol assists in decreasing obesity comparable to simply going on a low calorie diet. Scientists proved that when mammals ingest high levels of resveratrol it stopped them from gaining weight, and to their surprise, it turned them into the equivalent of Olympic marathoners!

Resveratrol also suppressed estrogen secretion. Keeping estrogen levels low contributes to a reduction in body fat and an increase in the ability to gain lean muscle; which enhances your metabolism to burn more calories and fat (see Estrogen-Progesterone chapter).

Since resveratrol suppresses estrogen, your testosterone levels will get that slight boost that can assist in burning extra fat and gain more muscle. This is great for men because it shrinks the undesired beer belly and increases the ever-so beloved muscle mass. But women should listen up too; we are often single-mindedly focused to lose those extra 10 pounds, and a small boost in testosterone levels this could very well be the key to success. As covered many times in this book…women should not be frightened about gaining muscle. Muscle will help you burn more calories throughout the day and also help us appear harder, leaner, and sexier! You will also lose extra fat. Put those two pieces together and you have a formula for a confidence booster.

Here are some of the encouraging affects you can achieve by supplementing with resveratrol:
Resveratrol is all-natural, safe, and comes from food.
Feel younger and stronger from antioxidants.
Increases fat loss.
Increases lean muscle mass.
Increases metabolism.
Helps treat and prevent diabetes through increased insulin sensitivity and lower blood glucose.
Prevents obesity.
Helps prevent cellular damage caused by free radicals; especially important for athletes!
Helps prevent retinopathy, which causes blindness and kidney failure.
Helps prevent heart disease, heart attacks, and stroke.
Helps prevent and control inflammation…the true cause of high cholesterol and clogged arteries!
Helps prevent the development and spread of cancer cells.
Reduces the risk of developing blood clots.
Supports the immune and autoimmune systems in fighting off disease.
Decreases pain and soreness due to arthritis.
Helps prevent the onset of Alzheimer's.
There are no undesired or unsafe side-effects.

With all this information about Resveratrol, I am a true believer of this antioxidant.

Supplement #4: L-CARNITINE: Fat Burner!

There is no doubt that the most effective means of attaining weight loss is by means of maintaining a well-balanced diet program and having a regular exercising routine. A very effective weight loss supplement that can be used alongside is carnitine which is extremely beneficial in increasing weight loss by mobilizing fat in the body and increasing calorie burning. Discovered in 1905, it is a water-soluble, vitamin-like compound that is readily used in the body. Dietary carnitine can be found in a number of foods. The best source is meat, particularly beef, sheep, and lamb. Other animal foods such as cheese and poultry contain somewhat less carnitine.

The function of carnitine is a bit complex. It is an amino acid which aids the breakdown of calories by shuttling fatty acids into the mitochondria which is our 'fat-burning powerhouse' in our body. The American Chronicle states there is also another significant reason which makes carnitine stand out among the various other weight loss supplements. Carnitine has the unique distinction of keeping watch and restricting the accumulation of fat around the liver and heart.

This unique supplement also helps enhance muscle strength and aids in reduction of triglyceride levels in the body. Carnitine furthermore helps reduce irritability and anxiety which is a common side effect amongst dieters. This supplement can help increase your energy at same time suppressing your appetite. Also muscular fatigue is reduced, which can help you go longer and harder in your fitness routine.

Nutrition rich foods and animal protein can help to meet basic levels of nutrition in the body. A person who exercises regularly needs lot of carnitine for overall growth and development. One should replenish this supplement in the body before a deficiency is created. Carnitine is suggested by doctors to those who don't consume adequate amounts of proteins, vitamins, and amino acids to make up for the deficiency. Deficiency of carnitine can lead to low energy levels and muscular weakness. Cramps and sudden weight gain are often a side effect of low levels of carnitine. Cardiovascular diseases, diabetes, Alzheimer's and obesity are some of the diseases which can occur if long term deficiency of carnitine happens. Due to lack of animal protein in the diet of vegetarians they are most likely to suffer from a deficiency. Doctors consider it to be a very effective supplement for vegetarians.

In the past carnitine was thought to be involved only in the conversion of fat into energy, but scientists have since discovered that it has many far-reaching actions critically related to your appearance, performance and overall health and longevity. Carnitine has been proposed by doctors and scientists as a treatment for many conditions. Here are some of the many benefits:

Weight Loss

L-Carnitine is one of the best supplements in the weight-loss industry which can help you lose those extra pounds. This supplement is most effective because it mobilizes the fat and it disappears more rapidly when you include it with your exercise program. Carnitine shuttles our extra fat to our fat-burning powerhouse in our cells called the mitochondria; energy is produced which enables you to burn fat easier and go longer during your workout. 2 grams before a workout on an empty stomach produces the best results.

Exercise Performance and aging

Aging results in deterioration of the muscles, an increase in body fat, and a decrease in our muscle's oxidative abilities. One study fed old rats with carnitine at 30 mg/kg body weight, the carnitine levels and oxidative activity of muscle cells was restored. Body composition was also improved; it decreased their abdominal fat and increased muscle fibers. Another study found L-carnitine in a dose of 100 mg/kg body weight improved exercise endurance.

Carnitine has strong antioxidant effects in the body, protecting cell membranes against free radical damage, which occurs at high rates during exercise and as part of the normal aging process. Therefore, long-term carnitine supplementation may slow the detrimental effects of aging on athletic performance.

Hyperthyroidism

Some research suggests that carnitine may prove useful for preventing or reducing symptoms of an overactive thyroid, such as insomnia, nervousness, elevated heart rate, and tremors. In fact, in one study, a small group of people with hyperthyroidism had improvement in these symptoms, as well as normalization of their body temperature, when taking carnitine.

Heart Conditions

- **Angina** -- The top facts for carnitine's use for heart disease is as an addition to conventional treatment for stable angina. Several clinical trials indicate that carnitine can help reduce symptoms of angina and improve the ability of those with angina to exercise without chest pain. You should not self-treat chest pain, however; see your doctor for diagnosis and conventional treatment, and consider carnitine as extra insurance for your heart.
- **Heart attack** -- Some studies suggest that people who take carnitine supplements soon after a heart attack may be less likely to suffer another heart attack, experience chest pain, or develop heart failure. Carnitine should be used along with conventional medication under your doctor's supervision.
- **Heart Failure** -- A few studies have found that carnitine (in the form of propionyl-L-carnitine) can help reduce symptoms of heart failure and improve exercise capacity in people with heart failure. However, more studies are needed to confirm any benefit.

Peripheral Vascular Disease

Decreased blood flow to the legs from atherosclerosis (plaque build-up) often causes an aching or cramping pain in the legs while walking or exercising. The reduced blood flow to the legs is called peripheral vascular disease. A number of studies show that carnitine can help ease symptoms and increase the distance people can walk. Most studies have used propionyl-L-carnitine; it isn't known if L-carnitine would have the same effect.

Diabetic Neuropathy

High blood sugar levels and diabetes often damage nerves in the body, especially the arms, legs, and feet; the condition is called diabetic neuropathy. Some studies suggest acetyl-L-carnitine may help decrease pain and increase normal feeling in affected nerves. It is also promising that carnitine can help nerves regenerate.

Male Infertility and Erectile Dysfunction

Low sperm counts have been connected to low carnitine levels. Numerous studies advocate that carnitine supplementation may enhance sperm count and motility. Studies also suggest that propionyl-L-carnitine could help male sexual function. One study found that carnitine significantly improved the effectiveness of Viagra in men with diabetes who until that time had not responded to Viagra.

Chronic Fatigue Syndrome (CFS)

Scientists find that chronic fatigue syndrome may be causes by deficiencies of many nutrients, including carnitine. L-carnitine has been compared to a medication for fatigue in a study of 30 people with CFS. Those who took carnitine did much better than those who took the medication, particularly after receiving the supplement for 4 - 8 weeks.

DOSAGE RECOMMENDATION

- Weight loss: 2 - 4 grams daily
- Peripheral vascular disease: 2 - 4 g per day
- Diabetic neuropathy: 3 g per day
- Male infertility: 500 - 1,000 mg three times daily
- Chronic fatigue syndrome: 500 - 1,000 mg up to four times per day
- Overactive thyroid: 2 - 4 g per day in two to four divided doses

Supplement #5: Co-Enzyme Q10

CoQ10 is one of the most essential supplements required by the body to maintain and enhance our shape. Co-enzyme Q10 is an antioxidant nutrient found in each and every cell of the body. This antioxidant helps the body produce energy within each cell. The "powerhouse" of cellular energy is the mitochondria. The mitochondrion is where fat-burning takes place. The more CoQ10 we have, the more mitochondria; therefore more fat-burning. Working together with the other metabolic supplements; such as l-carnitine, green tea, and alpha-lipoic acid, CoQ10 increases metabolism, providing greater energy, endurance, and ability to lose body fat, while preventing the energy decline seen in aging cells. It also assists in weight loss by regulating blood sugar, enhancing insulin sensitivity and maximizing the movement of fats in our blood to be used for fuel.

COQ10 VS ADVIL:
Patients have more than 50% reduction in the number of days with migraine headaches while using COQ10.

Hundreds of studies document the effectiveness of CoQ10 in protecting all vital organs of the body, including the brain, heart, and kidneys. Because of its powerful anti-inflammatory effects, CoQ10 is extremely protective of the cardiovascular system. It keeps the heart muscle healthy and also prevents inflammation in the arteries, which leads to arteriosclerosis. The ability of co-enzyme Q10 to effectively pump blood to your heart leaves you with immense energy. Also the viscosity of blood is lowered which improves the efficiency of heart.

This supplement also boosts your immune system. The ability of your body to deal with diseases is increased because the level of antibodies also increases. It prevents gum diseases by enabling the healing power of your gums thus giving them an ultimate strength. Co-enzyme q10 is very helpful for weight loss, multiple sclerosis, high blood pressure, diabetes, chronic fatigue, muscle weakness and muscular dystrophy.

According to Adam Russell, PhD, a human-performance expert, long-term CoQ10 supplementation may help athletes to recover more quickly after high-intensity workouts. A 2008 study published in the

Journal of the International Society of Sports Nutrition reported that 14 days of CoQ10 increased trained athletes' time to exhaustion in an endurance exercise test.

Although CoQ10 can be found in small amounts in fish such as sardines or salmon, as well as in nuts, supplementation is best for anti-aging and weight-loss. CoQ10 supplementation is of particular importance for women because they tend to have lower levels than men.

COQ10 TIPS

- This supplement should be taken by anyone over 40, as tissue levels of CoQ10 decrease as people get older.
- CoQ10 is best absorbed when taken with food including fat.
- Minimum of 60 mg per day up to 400 mg per day. About three weeks of daily dosing are necessary to reach maximal serum concentrations of CoQ10.

Supplement #6 Alpha Lipoic Acid (ALA)

Alpha Lipoic Acid is a powerful antioxidant and anti-inflammatory, both water- and fat-soluble. Because alpha lipoic acid is found only in trace amounts in food, it must be taken as a supplement. Alpha lipoic acid is found naturally in the body, inside the part of the cell called the mitochondria. It is closely involved in the energy production of the cell. Alpha lipoic acid, like many of the other nutrients including L-carnitine and CoQ10, enhances our ability to metabolize food into energy.

Unlike many other antioxidants such as vitamin C, which is strictly water soluble, or vitamin E, which is strictly fat soluble, alpha lipoic acid is soluble in both water and fat. This means that alpha lipoic acid can go to all parts of the cell, including fat portions such as the cell plasma membrane, as well as the interior of the cell where water-soluble pieces live. Because of this distinct ability, alpha lipoic acid is often called "the universal antioxidant." ALA also works with CoQ10 and l-carnitine to defend and restore the mitochondria. An aging cell is known to have a reduced energy production. The significance that ALA can boost energy levels in the cell and repair cells in the way that youthful cells do is extremely interesting.

Alpha lipoic acid also enhances the body's ability to get glucose into the cells; helping decrease our blood sugar levels. This insulin-sensitizing effect is also seen in L carnitine and other supplements discussed in this chapter. An increase in insulin sensitivity helps slow the aging and speed up the recovery process. ALA is a great supplement for anyone dealing with diabetes.

ALPHA LIPOIC ACID TIPS

- Assisting in our metabolism, alpha lipoic acid acts as a coenzyme in the production of energy by converting carbohydrates into energy; athletes may recognize this as ATP.
- ALA is the only antioxidant that can enhance levels of glutathione; which is our most important antioxidant to health and youth.
- Best absorption if taken with meals.

Supplement #7 CONJUGATED LINOLEIC (CLA)

CLA (Conjugated Linoleic Acid) helps convert fat to lean muscle mass. It is a fatty acid that is found in some of the foods we eat. At one time, beef, turkey, lamb and dairy were exceptional sources; however, when we changed their diet from grass to grains, the levels of CLA dramatically decreased in meat and dairy products. If CLA is present, it is found in the fatty portion of milk. Drinking skim milk prevents us from receiving the benefits of CLA.

CLA not only reduces fat but also preserves the muscle tissues. The most amazing part is not that it makes fat cell smaller but it prevents a small cell from becoming fatter. A low calorie diet often helps a person lose weight for a short period, but once the cravings take over and the diet comes to a halt, that person is even more likely to gain back the weight. Conjugated Linoleic Acid seems to stop this undesired weight gain from happening because it causes you to hold onto valuable muscles during weight loss. Studies show that CLA is also helpful in lowering blood sugar levels. In one study almost 2/3 of the volunteers had a reduction of blood glucose level and triglyceride levels.

This supplement helps in reducing fat at a faster rate. At least 3.4 grams per day must be taken in order for it to show its effect in our body.

It has been shown in numerous studies that people taking this supplement have around 6 pounds of weight lose as compared to others.

When taken in effective doses, CLA decreases body fat, especially in the area of the abdomen. Various studies prove the following additional benefits:

1. It can increase the rate of metabolism and is evidently very beneficial for thyroid patients.
2. People suffering from high cholesterol level and triglycerides can use this to lower levels at a faster rate.
3. It can also increase the growth of muscles which we now know stimulates our metabolism.
4. Many people suffer from the serious issue of insulin resistance in which CLA can be used to lower this resistance and therefore assist in controlling weight.
5. It can decrease Adrenal imbalances, which decreases abdominal fat stores.
6. It can help calm hormonal shifts; an area of concern to thyroid patients.
7. CLA has a very positive effect on our body by enhancing our immune system.

CLA TIPS

- When taken with sesame seeds, the effects of CLA are enhanced.
- The average diet provides minimal amounts of CLA, especially if eating low-fat dairy.
- CLA should be taken with meals.

DOSAGE RECOMMENDATION:

- 1000 mg, up to a maximum of 4000 mg per day, taken in one or two doses.

Glutamine is a particularly important supplement for anyone wanting to lose weight. Glutamine is mainly stored within muscles and is the body's most abundant amino acid. Amino acids are the basic building blocks of a protein. It's my favorite supplement and one I take pretty much all the time. It is an amazing supplement that helps a variety of people; the dieter, the workout warrior, the chronically ill, people with stomach and intestinal issues, cancer patients, and those recovering from surgery should be taking regularly. While most of the glutamine we need is produced in our muscles, we can also acquire a small amount of glutamine from dietary sources, such as poultry, fish, dairy products, and legumes.

Glutamine is extra important to those who exercise. It is used up very quickly during prolonged and intense cardiovascular workouts, such as running and aerobics and our body cannot make as much as it needs. This is bad because it causes the body to burn muscle for energy, exhausting our glutamine supply even further. Glutamine supplements enhance your body's ability to recover and stay healthy. After intense exercise your body's immune system is in a weakened condition making you more vulnerable to infections and disease. Glutamine supplements are recommended to take within 5 minutes after completing a workout or as soon as possible to give your muscles the best chance to become the lean, mean, fat burning machines we want them to be.

Glutamine has three main factors that increase athletic performance. The first is its ability to rebuild muscle tissue. This doesn't directly make them bigger, it allows for the muscles to recover faster resulting in a better workout next time. The more you can continue to challenge your body with exercise the better your results will be. The second part is that glutamine supports our body's ability to reload our muscles with nutrients. This directly relates to your muscles ability to increase lean body tissue, raising our metabolism. The third important piece for athletes is that it increases our human growth hormone output; which is our fat-burning hormone.

Glutamine is extremely helpful in the prevention of muscle breakdown caused by intense stress, physical injury, severe burns, disease, overexertion, poor nutrition, and dieting. Glutamine is extra special because it is the only amino acid that contains two nitrogen molecules. This additional molecule takes the nitrogen to where it is needed most. Nitrogen is one of the building blocks of muscle cells and glutamine is the delivery system for getting the nitrogen to those cells. Glutamine can also transport excess nitrogen out of the body; which is important because nitrogen can act as a toxin. The most favorable condition for muscle growth is when glutamine is working appropriately, and nitrogen intake is greater than nitrogen output.

Being overweight and having a body in an inflammatory state makes glutamine supplementation even more important. When the body is inflamed it breaks down the muscle tissue to get the extra glutamine it needs and this results in muscle loss. Getting extra glutamine allows the body to lose weight and retain muscle mass.

Glutamine is also very therapeutic for our digestive system. Intestinal health is important because it is the transport of fuel and nutrients. Glutamine is the fuel and nourishes the cells that line the digestive track and intestines. Time and time again studies have shown that a therapeutic dose of supplemental glutamine protects against aspirin-induced gastric lesions and helps heal painful ulcers. In fact, an old folk remedy for ulcers is cabbage juice, which is very high in glutamine. Stomach problems, such as colitis and Crohn's disease can be calmed by glutamine. Glutamine can be used whenever there are any stomach problems, as simple as drinking too much alcohol (alcoholic-induced gastritis) to ulcers, diarrhea, or even more serious problems such as inflammatory bowel disease.

Glutamine is also beneficial for a variety of other health issues.

1. Studies also find that glutamine will reduce cravings for high-glycemic carbohydrates and can make your weight-loss plan a lot easier.
2. Glutamine can help prevent both depression and fatigue and can also help us create neurotransmitters in the brain, which help relax us while elevating our mood. In the brain, it is transformed to glutamic acid and boosts the amount of GABA (gamma-aminobutyric acid). Both glutamic acid and GABA are considered "brain fuel," because they are necessary for everyday mental function.

3. Many studies have also found that therapeutic amounts of glutamine helps prevent the harmful effects of alcohol on the brain and may also decrease alcohol (as well as sugar) cravings.
4. It is also essential to our immune system, because it is utilized by white blood cells. Glutamine is now used in some hospitals intravenously to speed up recovery of patients. The better you develop your muscles through exercise, the more glutamine they produce which is one of the reasons fit people get sick less often.

DOSAGE RECOMMENDATION:

A recent study published by The American Journal of Clinical Nutrition has shown that oral supplementation with as little as 2 grams of glutamine significantly enhanced patients overall health!

Glutamine is considered a safe substance. Dosages of up to 21 grams a day have been demonstrated to have no negative side effects. High glutamine levels also support brain function, including better alertness. Taking 2 grams before bed increases human growth hormone. Recommended dosage is 5-20 grams a day for optimal health.

Supplement #9: 5-HTP: Dr. Oz's miracle cure!

Anxiety, depression, and obesity are issues I see every day with clients, each reinforcing the other. They don't understand why they feel the way they do and want to "snap out of it." Our brain biochemistry plays a huge part in our moods; which can drive us to unhealthy eating behaviors. A nutritional supplement called 5-HTP (5-hydroxy-L-tryptophan) has been a miracle cure for my clients. According to scientist Michael Murray, N.D., "Numerous double-blind studies have shown 5-HTP to be as effective as antidepressant drugs, but it is better tolerated and is associated with fewer and much milder side effects. The body converts tryptophan, an amino acid (protein) found in food, into 5-HTP, which is used to make serotonin; an important brain chemical regulating mood, behavior, appetite, and sleep."

In Europe, 5-HTP has been used for decades as a standard treatment for depression, sleep problems, weight loss, and other medical problems. It is now starting to be used in the USA. Scientific studies find that 5-HTP is a safe, natural way to increase the brain serotonin levels, which drop during dieting and when women menstruate (hence low moods, cravings and sleep issues...PMS). Interestingly, 5-HTP has been found to produce **results equal to or better than** those of standard synthetic drugs used in the problems arising from serotonin deficiency or depression. Dr. Ray Sahelian, M.D., author of "5-HTP: Nature's Serotonin Solution," believes 5-HTP holds a great deal of promise. He states, "5-HTP helps control appetite, improve mood, and reduce anxiety." Sounds good to me, sign me up!

HOW DOES 5-HTP WORK?

Mood and sleep disorders are imbalances in monoamine neurotransmitters. Having low levels of serotonin is an acknowledged factor in depression, obesity, and anxiety. Serotonin is a monoamine compound, chemically related to amino acid derivatives such as 5-HTP. This supplement also increases levels of endorphins and many other neurotransmitters, which help decrease our recurrence of depression and low moods.

When levels of serotonin fall, your body senses starvation. To protect itself, your body starts to crave carbohydrates. Serotonin levels fall after you go too long without eating and when estrogen levels fall during menstruation which encourages your body to start filling itself. People who use 5-HTP to keep their serotonin level up have more positive experience when dieting. Dr. Oz's book, "YOU! On a Diet," had a six-week study of 5-HTP and dieters. The group of dieters using 5-HTP lost an average of 12 pounds, while a control group lost an average of four. Ninety percent of women taking at least 300mg of 5-HTP report satiety while on a diet.

Fat Burning Tip:
Irony of Antidepressants:
Weight gain is a common side effect with many antidepressants and mood stabilizer medications. All antidepressants have the potential to cause weight gain; most people are unaware that weight gain is one of the most common side effects associated with Zoloft, Paxil, Prozac, Zyprexa and many other behavioral drugs until it is too late. Ironically, this common side effect causes an increase in depression as it can seriously impact self-esteem. 5-HTP is a natural antidepressant that can actually help decrease cravings to assist in weight loss.

Pharmaceutical antidepressants, like Prozac, Zoloft and Paxil, work by blocking the reabsorption of serotonin after it has performed its messenger function between nerve cells. These drugs, called SSRIs (selective serotonin re-uptake inhibitors) produce considerable unpleasant side effects, and **do not work effectively unless the body is producing sufficient levels of serotonin in the first place. Vegetarians are often lacking enough amino acids to produce serotonin.**

There have been controlled scientific studies comparing 5-HTP to an SSRI drugs, in most cases fluvoxamine, also known as Luvox and the drug Prozac. The participants receiving 5-HTP were found to have experienced a slightly better and faster relief than those who were given fluvoxamine, and a larger percentage of them had a positive reaction to 5-HTP. One study found that even though their serotonin levels increased, one in five participants who responded positively to 5-HTP relapses after one month because levels of other brain chemicals, also known as monamines decreased. These patients responded terrifically to additional supplementation with the amino acid tyrosine. I use a product that has both 200mg of 5-HTP and 100mg of l-tyrosine for these clients.

5-HTP and Obesity

Three clinical studies using a placebo and 5-HTP established that 5-HTP can be successful in assisting weight loss in overweight patients. It helps by creating feelings of satiety. People taking 5-HTP lost 3-5 times as much weight as those who were taking a placebo.

5-HTP and Insomnia

5- HTP provides the fastest, most effective, and most unfailing results in treating insomnia. It is an effective alternative for people suffering with sleep issues. It is a safe and natural supplement compared to prescription and over-the-counter sleep medicines. Prescription sleep medications slow metabolism. 5-HTP improves the quality of sleep as compared to most over-the-counter and pharmaceutical medications which knock you out but don't increase REM sleep; which is the quality sleep we are looking for. 5-HTP increases REM sleep by about 25 percent, while at the same time as increasing deep sleep stages 3 and 4 without increasing total sleep time. 5-HTP accomplishes this by shortening the amount of time you spend in sleep stages 1 and 2, which are the least important stages sleep. The higher the dose, the more time spent in REM. By shifting the balance of the sleep cycle, 5-HTP makes sleep more restful and rejuvenating. Instead of waking feeling just as tired and "hung-over," as many people experience with medications like Tylenol PM, people taking 5- HTP feel energetic and well-rested. When we get quality sleep, we dream more efficiently and wake up with our physical and mental batteries fully charged. The effectiveness of 5-HTP on sleep stages is dose-related; taking higher doses generates a greater impact, but usually a lower dose is sufficient. Higher doses may create more dreams or nightmares due to abnormally long REM sleep.

5-HTP and Headaches

Scientific studies find that 5-HTP is as successful as pharmaceutical drugs in decreasing symptoms of migraine headaches, because of the increase in serotonin.

DOSAGE RECOMMENDATIONS

- 100 up 500mg per night
- My favorite dose: NOW Brand carries...200mg 5-HTP with 100mg l-tyrosine. I recommend 2 of these before bed.
- NOTE: Do not take with prescription anti-depressants

Supplement #10: GABA – decrease anxiety

Anxiety and depression may be the result of shortages of key brain neurotransmitters, one of which is called GABA, which can be restored naturally. Give the brain the amino acids it needs and feel your mind start to glow again.

If you're one of the millions who suffer from anxiety or depression, the next time you reach for the Valium or Prozac; consider amino acids as a safe alternative. These protein building blocks may be the key to reversing long-standing anxiety and depression, according to Harold Whitcomb, M.D., and biochemical nutritionist Phyllis Bronson. They regularly prescribe amino acids for their clients at the Aspen, Colorado Clinic for Preventive and Environmental Medicine.

Mood, behavior, and brain biochemistry are intricately linked. Depression and anxiety may be the result of flawed message-sending in the brain, flawed because key brain chemicals called neurotransmitters are in short supply. They're short because the body's amino acid pool, from which they're made, is itself low. For example, deficiencies in the amino acid GABA are strongly correlated with states of anxiety. Add this to the negative effect of high levels of heavy metals commonly found in the body. Aluminum, mercury, lead, and copper can make the body toxic, interfere with brain function, and contribute to depression and anxiety.

For 90% of dieters, a deficiency in one of four key brain chemicals can trigger weight gain, fatigue, and stress. The key to losing weight doesn't lie in deprivation diets; it lies in balancing our neurochemicals. Many nutritionists and advanced practitioners are focusing on how the brain affects our health.

1. Dopamine controls metabolism
2. Acetylcholine regulates fat storage
3. GABA curbs emotional eating
4. Serotonin influences appetite.

When these primary brain chemicals are balanced, our bodies are more able to lose those unwanted pounds.

Increase the amino acids that make up with the missing neurotransmitters, and flush the toxic metals out of the body, and you start seeing dramatic improvements in both depression and anxiety, report Whitcomb and Bronson. "By using supplements of the amino acids that make up specific neurotransmitters, you can actually change the nature and intensity of the brain messages they carry and thus the emotions they affect."

Even better, you don't get the serious side effects commonly associated with pharmaceutical medications. These can typically include a decrease in metabolism, blurred vision, increased heart rate, low blood pressure, nausea, headaches, constipation, memory loss, impaired concentration, and brain fog. In contrast, the clinical use of amino acids produces no side effects or health risks and generates better, more lasting healing results, says Bronson. Bronson has been studying this for 20 years; it is called orthomolecular medicine and was first established in the 1950's.

THE SCIENCE OF BRAIN CHEMICALS

Patients typically have positive results in 3 to 4 weeks, Bronson reports, but in acute cases, there is often a significant improvement in a matter of days. Many patients who come to the clinic are on powerful drugs called psychotropics, which include Valium and Prozac, to control their anxiety or depression. The goal is to increase the patient's amino acid reserves so they can eventually discontinue these drugs. However, this is not possible or advisable in all cases, so then the goal is to reduce the potential toxicity of the psychotropics which will often reduce the side effects. It all comes down to brain chemicals. "When people take Prozac for depression, they're actually trying to biochemically elevate their serotonin levels." Bronson states. "When people take Valium and the other benzodiazepene drugs for anxiety, they're trying to elevate their GABA levels." People with deficiencies in serotonin tend to be depressed while people without enough GABA suffer anxiety. "What we do is substitute the natural neurotransmitters or their amino acid precursors for the psychotropic drugs." The result is more thorough healing with no side effects.

The first step in reversing anxiety and depression is to see which factors are at play. For example, there may be a genetic factor involved in which a person is somewhat predisposed at birth to be lacking in a specific neurotransmitter. Inadequate diet and nutrition is another factor that can leave one's system deficient in key minerals. The stress of today's fast-paced lifestyle may also deplete the body's reserves of amino acids and vital nutrients. One of Bronson's clients had an undiagnosed toxic response to baked potatoes, which she ate every day thinking they were good for her. Some people have brain allergies to foods they eat regularly, and these can show up like depression when it's actually a chronic food allergy response instead.

Natural ways to correct the biochemical pathways associated with anxiety and depression are by elevating levels of key nutrients called amino acids; which are precursors to the neurotransmitters. Then the body does the rest on its own. In most cases, about 50% of people require an ongoing maintenance level of amino acids to keep their anxiety or depression under control, while others are able to eventually discontinue them.

The use of amino acids rather than pharmaceutical medicine seems to empower, even motivate, people to get well. People who take nutrients under proper guidance seem to have a sense of power over what's happening to them whereas many people taking pharmaceutical medications often feel that they're surrendering to some mystery that is quite upsetting.

Mind and body overlap in a complex biochemistry of neurotransmitter pathways. Gaba is just one piece of the puzzle that can help patients heal depression and anxiety naturally.

DOSAGE RECOMMENDATIONS

- Up to 500 mg 3 times daily on an empty stomach
- 1 gram before bed can increase human growth hormone

Supplement #11: Magnesium

What mineral is needed by every cell in the body, yet odds are you don't get enough of it? Hint: It's not calcium. Give up? It's magnesium. It gets little attention now, but rising evidence implies that magnesium benefits your heart and bones, plus it may help prevent diabetes and migraine headaches. Magnesium is the fourth most abundant mineral in the body and is vital to a healthy body. Roughly 50% of total body magnesium is found in bone. The other half is found inside the cells of body tissues and organs.

Magnesium is essential for more than 300 biochemical actions in the body. Magnesium is vital for healthy aging and disease prevention. Studies have shown that magnesium deficiencies correlate to Alzheimer's and Parkinson's. Deficiencies also cause muscle spasms, pain, insomnia and fatigue. Magnesium assists in maintaining muscle mass, nerve function, a regular heart beat, helps our immune system, and keeps bones strong. Diabetics benefit from magnesium as it helps regulate blood sugar levels. In addition, it normalizes blood pressure, and is known to be involved in energy metabolism and protein synthesis. There has been a lot of medical interest in using magnesium to avoid and manage disorders such as cardiovascular disease, diabetes, and hypertension.

The health of our digestive system and the kidneys is jeopardized if we are deficient in magnesium. This mineral is absorbed in the intestines and then transported through the blood into the cells and tissues. Gastrointestinal disorders such as Crohn's disease or a food allergy can limit the body's ability to absorb magnesium. These disorders can deplete the body's stores of magnesium and in extreme cases may result in magnesium deficiency. Chronic vomiting and diarrhea will also deplete magnesium levels. Alcohol abuse and uncontrolled diabetes are other causes of magnesium deficiency.

Early signs of magnesium deficiency include nausea, fatigue, or weakness. As magnesium deficiency gets worse, migraines, restless leg syndrome, numbness, muscle cramps, seizures, mood changes, or irregular heartbeats can occur. Severe magnesium deficiency can also deplete the levels of calcium in the blood. Americans have the highest dietary intake of calcium in the world, yet we have the highest rate of hip fractures…hmmm, could a magnesium deficiency be the cause? Magnesium deficiency is also associated with low levels of potassium in the blood.

Magnesium is also being researched as a natural way to curb food cravings. It is found that as magnesium deficiencies increase so do food cravings. **Supplementing with a therapeutic dose of 600milligrams of magnesium is a natural way to tame those unruly carbohydrate desires.**

Leafy green vegetables, nuts and seeds are good sources of magnesium. The chart below lists plenty of dietary sources of magnesium, but note that we should get at least 400mg of magnesium a day…are you getting enough?

FOOD Sources of Magnesium	Milligrams (mg)	%DV
Halibut, cooked, 3 ounces	90	20
Almonds, dry roasted, 1 ounce	80	20
Cashews, dry roasted, 1 ounce	75	20
Spinach, frozen, cooked, ½ cup	75	20
Nuts, mixed, dry roasted, 1 ounce	65	15
Peanuts or peanut butter, 1 ounce	50	15
Yogurt, plain, 8 fluid ounces	45	10
Avocado, California, ½ cup pureed	35	8

Eating a variety of nuts and dark-green leafy vegetables every day will help provide recommended intakes of magnesium and maintain normal storage levels of this mineral. However, increasing magnesium through food may not be enough to restore extremely low magnesium levels to normal. Oral therapeutic doses of magnesium supplements in the form of magnesium-citrate or magnesium-glycinate is the best way to ensure proper levels.

Health Benefits: Magnesium
-Aids in fighting depression
-Reduces food cravings
-Beneficial in the treatment of PMS
-Relieves restless leg syndrome
-Particularly important for maintaining a normal heart rhythm and is often used by physicians to treat irregular heartbeat or arrhythmia.
-Beneficial for bladder problems in women, especially common disturbances in bladder control and the sense of "urgency."
-Lowers blood pressure
-Beneficial in the treatment of neuromuscular and nervous disorders
-Prevents kidney stones and gallstones
-Vital for a healthy immune system
-Keeps teeth healthy
-Magnesium is used by the body to help maintain muscles, nerves, and bones
-Energy metabolism and protein synthesis
-Helps regulate blood sugar levels
-Useful in treatment of polio and post-polio syndrome
-Useful in the treatment of prostate problems
-Helps reduce stress

Muscle building

Magnesium supplements are often times marketed as muscle enhancers and testosterone boosters. Magnesium is a natural muscle relaxant; which is extremely helpful for rebuilding our tired overused muscles. If you are strength training...I hope you are...then supplementing with magnesium before bed will help your muscles repair faster for the next day's feats. Athletes also run the risk of having a lower immune system because your body is more focused on your muscles, but adding magnesium can significantly boost you immune system during times of serious exercise.

Premenstrual syndrome

Increasing evidence shows premenstrual syndrome might also be triggered by dietary deficiencies in certain vitamins or minerals, especially magnesium. Magnesium deficiency has direct correlation as a factor in premenstrual syndrome. Magnesium levels in PMS patients have been shown to be significantly lower than in normal subjects. Many women with PMS have high sugar intakes, which lower magnesium values in the blood. Supplemental magnesium appears to be a great natural cure.

Blood pressure

Recent studies find that magnesium may play an important role in regulating blood pressure. The DASH study (Dietary Approaches to Stop Hypertension); a human clinical trial, suggested that high blood pressure could be significantly lowered by a diet high in magnesium, potassium, and calcium. Diets filled with nuts and vegetables, which are good sources of potassium and magnesium, are without fail linked to lower blood pressure.

A study examined the effect of various nutritional factors on incidence of high blood pressure in over 30,000 US male health professionals. After four years, it was found that a lower risk of hypertension was associated with increased amounts of magnesium, potassium, and dietary fiber. A 6-year study of 8,000 patients who were initially free of hypertension, found that the risk of developing hypertension increases if a magnesium deficiency occurred.

Diabetes

Diabetes is the result of insufficient production or use of insulin. Insulin converts sugar and starches in our diet into energy. Magnesium plays a significant function in carbohydrate metabolism by assisting the release and activity of insulin. A magnesium deficiency aggravates insulin resistance, a condition that starts the ball rolling for diabetes, and deficiencies are commonly found in patients with type 2 diabetes. Kidneys possibly lose their ability to maintain magnesium levels during periods of elevated levels of blood glucose. Magnesium is lost during the increased urination. Supplementing with a therapeutic dose of magnesium may improve insulin levels.

Cardiovascular disease

Magnesium influences metabolism, diabetes, and high blood pressure; all of which increases the probability that magnesium influences cardiovascular disease. Extended surveys have connected higher blood levels of magnesium with lower risk of heart disease. Some dietary surveys also found that higher magnesium levels may reduce the risk of having a stroke. Evidence also proves that low levels of magnesium increase the risk of abnormal heart rhythms, which adds to the risk of complications after a heart attack.

Researchers studied the effects of magnesium supplementation and the ability to walk on a treadmill, chest pain caused by exercise, and quality of life. Patients received either a therapeutic dose of 400 milligrams of magnesium-citrate twice daily for 6 months or a placebo. At the end of the study period researchers found that magnesium therapy significantly improved magnesium levels. Patients receiving magnesium had a 14 percent improvement in exercise duration and experienced less chest pain caused by exercise as compared to no change in the placebo group.

RECOMMENDED DOSE

Dietary magnesium does not pose a health risk, however therapeutic doses of magnesium in supplements can promote unfavorable effects such as diarrhea. Choosing the correct form of magnesium will help prevent this undesired effect. Magnesium oxide is found in Milk of Magnesia…so of course that version of magnesium will cause diarrhea. Choose magnesium-citrate or magnesium-glycinate; these are highly absorbable forms and cannot be found in your typical retail store. Talk to your local health food store, nutritionist or chiropractor. These versions are a little more expensive, but you are ensuring absorption of the nutrient; it is money well spent.

I recommend taking 400mg to 800mg of magnesium around 30 minutes before going to bed. Someone suffering from migraines or takes medication that depletes magnesium, they may require more; up to 1,000mg per day. Magnesium is a natural muscle relaxant that improves sleep. In addition to supplements, taking baths with magnesium salts provides added benefits. Absorbing magnesium through the skin stimulates the production of DHEA, the anti-aging hormone.

Supplement #12 Probiotics

Did you know that our moods stem from our gut? Yep, our nerve endings run from our intestines to our brain. Low good bacteria equals low serotonin, which cause low moods, cravings and sleep issues.

An interesting issue with the struggle to lose weight is gut bacterial overgrowth. Unfortunately, there is an alarming misconception about bacterial overgrowth in our country. The problem is not only with an overgrowth of bad bacteria, but too much bacteria in general. **Recent studies uncovered the additional functions of bacteria in our bodies. One example demonstrates that bacteria helps us to survive in times of famine by extracting extra calories from our food that would normally be burned off during normal digestion, and storing them as fat.** I don't think any of us have to worry about starving to death anytime soon.

Good bacteria known as probiotics are helpful micro-organisms that live in our intestinal tract. In a healthy body, good bacteria make up most of the intestines' micro-flora and protect digestive health. If you have primarily good bacteria, your immune system will function optimally and it will help you extract essential nutrients in the foods you eat.

Bacterial overgrowth can be a result of antibiotics, other medications, colonics, colonoscopies, stress, poor diet, over-consumption of yeast, low stomach acid, caffeine and alcohol. People with poor intestinal flora often suffer from intestinal discomfort, yeast infections, Candida overgrowth, constipation, bloating, and weight gain. Reintroducing probiotics quickly normalizes digestive health, prevents infections, strengthens the immune system, and helps you lose weight. Treating bacteria overgrowth depends on the severity; adding probiotics and changing your diet will help with mild cases. This sounds easy, but depriving yourself of your favorite foods can be challenging. Stay away from refined sugar and grains; fermented foods like beer, wine, and vinegar (mustards), yeast breads, and dried fruit. Severe overgrowth also may require a natural antimicrobial supplement such as Candex.

Probiotics are also found in the small intestine where they assist the body in multiple digestive and protective processes, including the absorption of minerals and vitamins; blocking of yeasts, harmful bacteria and viruses; such as salmonella, E.coli, Candida, and herpes. Probiotics can even neutralize cancer-causing toxins; which are produced by our bodies from nitrates and nitrites contained in processed meats and cigarette smoke.

Many practitioners prescribe probiotics to help obese people lose weight by stimulating their metabolism and killing destructive intestinal micro-organisms that contribute to a larger waistline. Recent studies have shown that helpful bacteria can metabolize complex carbohydrates, such as difficult-to-digest vegetables, therefore reducing bloating, accumulation of waste, and stomach pains which is typical when fiber consumption is increased.

If you are struggling with your weight and common gut issues; such as gas, bloating, indigestion, constipation, diarrhea, feeling full yet hungry or persistent skin problems you could be under attack with an overgrowth of bacteria. **Unless you take action to resolve the overgrowth of bacteria your body will resist to losing even an ounce of fat. The over-consumption of yeast is a major factor of weight gain and by taking a probiotic for weight loss will prevent the pounds from piling on.**

The most common probiotic for weight loss found today is called 'acidophilus' and is available in capsule form. These healthy bacteria can prevent digestive problems and is also known to help Crohn's disease sufferers. Probiotics for weight loss also helps the thyroid gland which in turn increases metabolism. This gives people with thyroid problems a much needed boost in shedding excess weight.

Bifido-bacteria is another helpful probiotic; which is found in the large intestine and colon. The main function of bifido is to inhibit the growth of bad bacteria and absorb the essential B-vitamins. Recent science shows that Bifido-bacteria also reduces "bad" cholesterol levels. Bifido is found in mother's breast milk and is essential for babies' digestion. If your baby is suffering from chronic stomach pains, adding bifido to a quality formula is extremely helpful.

Healthy indigenous people from various parts of the world always included bacteria-rich foods in their daily menu were consistently consumed by the lean Inuit, Masai, Maori, Russians, Norwegians, and many other early societies. The healthy bacteria produced trim bodies and superior health.

In order to get more probiotics in your diet, be it for weight-loss purposes or to improve intestinal health, you can get them from food sources, just as our ancestors did. Raw cheeses, properly-made unflavored yogurts, sauerkraut, and kombucha, are just a few examples of a vast array of probiotic-containing foods. I recommend that you eat small amount of sauerkraut or fermented veggies with your meals, to boost the immune system, improve digestion, and assist in shedding off excess weight. If you aren't a fan of

Food manufacturers quickly jumped on the bandwagon soon after scientists touted how essential good bacteria can be for weight loss. The market became flooded with "stomach-friendly" processed products, mainly yogurts containing "live bacteria". TV advertisements show active, happy, and slim women holding cups of probiotic yogurts. Yes, probiotics can help us lose weight, but not when it is mixed with a plastic container filled with high fructose corn syrup.

these foods, it is cheap and easy to add in a supplemental probiotic. I always take these after I need a round of antibiotics.

If you decide to take a probiotic for weight loss you should always use the most effective strain of probiotics which creates an environment that yeasts cannot survive in. Probiotics for weight loss in capsule form should always be stored in the fridge to prevent them from 'dying' and becoming useless. These probiotics in capsule form can be purchased from most health food stores or the internet but remember that they must be kept cool so ensure the postage time is not too long and that the storage facilities are adequate.

Digestive enzymes can play a big part in weight control and reveal a hidden factor in obesity. When most people hear the word enzyme, their mind drifts to digestion. Being imperfect humans, our digestive systems don't necessarily work to its capacity. For many people our bodies don't make enough of a certain enzyme, which results in an inability to properly digest food.

Although it is important to get adequate fluids throughout your day, drinking with meals can slow metabolism. Fluids dilute digestive enzymes in your stomach and can cause indigestion…beer is the worst culprit. So focus on your water consumption before and at least 30 minutes after meals.

Perhaps you've taken a digestive enzyme formula for indigestion. Supplemental enzymes are extremely helpful and natural ways to decrease gas, bloating, heartburn and indigestion. People often take enzymes for a few days, or even a few weeks, but then the bottle often goes back in the medicine cabinet or you go back to the antacids that so many people turn to, thanks to the marketing "geniuses". Enzymes primary task is digestion; however, they do so much more.

The enzyme guru, DicQui Fuller, defines enzymes as "proteins taken from food and made by the body." Every chemical reaction in our body relies on enzymes to be present; which means that every action our body does requires enzymes to perform it. Even vitamins, minerals, and hormones are unable to do their jobs without enzymes. Our body is lifeless without them.

Enzymes are extremely helpful in healthy weight loss. Lipase is an enzyme that is plentiful in foods that are raw and since very few of us have a diet rich in raw foods we lack sufficient amounts to burn normal amounts of fat in our diets. When you have enough lipase, your body is able to break down and dissolve the fat stored throughout the body. Without this essential enzyme, fat builds up and is stored in your arteries and around your organs; which harms us internally. Externally, fat starts to accumulate on hips, abdomen, our "bum", and thighs. Protease is another important enzyme which breaks down proteins and eliminates toxins. When your body carries toxins we become very inefficient in burning fat and fat is where our body stores extra toxins. Supplementing with protease will help eliminate toxins; which is why these two enzymes are so important when you are trying to lose weight.

If your body is lacking enzymes, it can't absorb all the nutrients from your diet. Your body receives a signal that it needs to store more fat against the threat of starvation. Our body is also told to take in more food to get more nutrients, causing intense cravings! A lack of enzymes creates a domino effect where we eat more and more, still always feeling hungry, still don't digest the nutrients we need, store more fat, and in that fat is more toxins. The right digestive enzyme formula can stop this undesired spiral of issues and help your body rebalance, as well as keeping cravings at bay.

Enzymes for weight loss can take some time. Adding therapeutic doses of supplemental enzymes for around three weeks, called the 'integration period,' is the first step. During the integration period, your appetite may swing back and forth considerably, as the body starts to adapt to absorb so much more nutrients from the foods you are eating and you also start a detoxification as the body breaks up rancid fats, toxic by-products, and undigested proteins of incomplete digestion. After the initial three weeks, another three to six weeks are typically required before we feel renewed energy and experience naturally occurring weight loss.

Enzymes are found in raw foods, but most of us cook our veggies, buy frozen or canned items that have been stripped from these important enzymes. Therefore supplemental enzymes are a good and cheap insurance for healthy elimination, absorption of essential nutrients, and regeneration of cells. Over time, enzymes will restore your energy and build stamina more than any other single supplement and this is another reason why they are so very helpful for weight loss.

If you are like most clients I see who are stressed out, don't get enough sleep, don't have enough time for frequent exercise, drink alcohol, and eat foods with additives your body's enzyme level becomes compromised. As we age we also produce fewer enzymes.

There are many different enzymes for specific nutrients. The main three that we should be aware of that will assist you in your weight loss goals are:

1. Protease, which helps break down protein
2. Amylase, which helps break down carbohydrates / sugars / starches
3. Lipase, which helps break down fats / lipids.

If you think about it, that's what everything we eat consists of......protein, carbohydrates, and fats. There are many products out there that combine all three so you don't need to take all of them separate. Therapeutic doses of these enzymes can help your body handle, break down, and digest what you are giving it, and better utilize it for what we really want to accomplish; burn unwanted body fat. So, try it out, it just might be what you need to take your weight loss to the next level.

Supplement #14 Whey Protein

Did you know that if you gain 10 pounds of muscle, you will burn an extra 3500 calories per week? To burn that many calories doing cardio, you'd have to run for an hour each day of the week! To build 10 pounds of muscle, feed your body a high quality whey protein drink 1-3 times a day, and increase strength training. Whey protein is my favorite addition to my diet in the past few years. It provides me with the muscle maintaining protein I need when I work out or don't consume the calories I need in a day.

Whey is a form of protein that is naturally-present in dairy products like milk, cottage cheese and yogurt. Two issues I often see in athletic clients are they either do so much cardio that they tear down their muscles which kills their metabolism or they dip too low in calories which eats up their valuable muscle for energy. Whey protein is a popular protein supplement for fitness fanatics mainly because of its high concentration in the branched chain amino acids (BCAAs), leucine, isoleucine, and valine. BCAAs are the key players in maintaining muscle tissue and help to preserve muscle stores of glycogen and can help prevent muscle protein breakdown during exercise; again…let's keep that metabolism humming. Consuming whey as a protein source for a post-exercise snack is awesome for our exhausted muscles.

Whey protein is also very low in fat and carbohydrates. This is because the refinement process used to create whey protein powder removes nearly all of the fat and sugars in the liquid, leaving a final product that is almost 100% protein by volume. This makes whey protein great for dieters who want to hold onto their valuable muscle. Athletes, fitness enthusiasts and vegetarians find that whey protein helps them attain specific training goals and enhanced energy levels.

Whey protein has other properties that have health benefits, including the presence of certain biologically active nutrients that enhance the immune system and even stave off muscle wasting.

Whey Protein Benefits:

✓ Whey Protein is not stored as fat as easily as carbohydrates.
✓ Whey Protein decreases your hunger between meals.
✓ Whey Protein helps strengthen your immune system.
✓ Whey Protein increases energy levels, especially during low-calorie dieting and helps shorten recovery time between exercise sessions.
✓ Whey Protein helps repair and build new muscle.

Each type of protein has a specific biological value. The higher the value, the better it works. Whey protein has the highest biological value (bv) of any protein, 104. Beef has a bv of 80 and soy protein with a bv of 74. That means whey protein is 23% more effective than beef and 29% more effective than soy protein at helping you body build lean muscle! Unlike other proteins, like casein, which is another form of protein in milk, the speed at which whey protein is digested makes it an ultimate source of protein following exercise when your body requires amino acids promptly to aid with recovery.

Top 10 reasons to consume WHEY:
1. **Boost Immune System** – Whey protein includes high levels of the amino acid cysteine, which produces glutathione, a potent antioxidant that maintains immune health. One of the first indications in patients with autoimmune diseases is a decrease in glutathione levels. Many studies have proven adding whey protein to patients with chronic fatigue syndrome, cancer, and HIV can greatly enhance their immune system. Scientists discovered that whey proteins stopped the growth of breast cancer cells in test tubes. It was also proven that when patients ingest at least 24 grams of whey a day they had a noteworthy reduction in the size of cancer tumors.

Top 10 reasons to consume WHEY:
2. Enhance Infant Formula– Whey protein contains alpha-lactalbumin and is the main nutrient in human breast milk. This makes whey protein a very important nutrient to include in infant formulas and should be the first protein consumed by babies. Good news to mothers, the Journal of Pediatrics, found that formulas with whey protein have been shown to help reduce the length of crying spells in babies with colic. Always check the ingredients list on your infant formula, not all contain whey because it costs more.
3. Benefit Cardiovascular Health –Adding whey along with your doctor's prescription can be a great balance to help your heart. Clinical research discovered that whey protein reduces blood pressure in individuals who are borderline hypertensive.
4. Increase Lean Body Mass– Our muscles need branched chain amino acids (BCAAs) during long periods of exercise and added stress; which can also have a negative effect on the immune system. Whey proteins are naturally high in BCAAs that are easy to digest. It immediately supplies the muscles with high quality protein it is screaming for; which directly correlates to an increase in physical performance and enhanced body composition.
5. Contribute to a Positive Mood– Stress is a well-known cause of a decrease in serotonin levels in the brain; which can cause depression. Clinical studies found that including whey protein is helpful in enhancing moods and in boosting serotonin levels because it is high in tryptophan, a natural relaxant. Whey is great for people with high stress lifestyles and elevated cortisol hormones.
6. Superior Protein Source for Lactose, Casein or Gluten Free Diets- Whey protein isolate is the purest form and is over 90% protein. Whey protein isolate contains only trace amounts of lactose, therefore people with lactose allergies can safely enjoy whey. It is also a great protein source for people with Celiac disease who are on gluten or wheat protein-restricted diets.
7. An Appetite Suppressor – One of the nutrients in whey protein, glycomacropeptide, stimulates the release of cholecystokinin, which is an appetite suppressing hormone.
8. Stave off Osteoporosis – Osteoporosis affects over 25 million Americans. We have the highest rate of hip fractures, yet we have the highest intake of calcium in the world, next to Sweden. Studies show that low protein intake, including low levels of animal protein consumption, was directly related to increased levels of bone loss. Impact exercise, such as walking, and sufficient amounts of protein in the diet can enhance bone health and may help to reduce the frequency of osteoporosis.
9. Help Protect against Ulcers and Acid Reflux – Lactoferrin, a nutrient in whey protein, is a known inhibitor of many forms of bacteria that is responsible for digestive problems; such as gastritis and ulcers. In addition, recent animal studies show promising results that it also kills the bacteria responsible for acid reflux.
10. Aid Wound Healing – People who have burns or are recovering from surgery require additional protein in their diet. Exciting new studies indicate whey protein nutrients promote the growth of new body tissue.

So calling whey an "ultimate protein" isn't too far off the mark. It supplies an easily digested, complete protein for reloading the muscles and enhances our health as a bonus! It has superior qualities over soy, rice and egg proteins. Adding whey into your diet is easy and flavorful.

Studies find the most beneficial time for athletes to include whey is during the post-workout "glycogen window," the 10 to 30 minute period immediately after exercising. This is when exhausted muscles are most interested to replacing depleted nutrients. Preparing a protein shake is quick and easy, and the liquid protein is digested immediately compared to a full meal. You'll gain muscle mass much more easily if you consume a protein mix immediately post-workout. Even if you're not hungry you should consume protein to hold onto muscle. Whey is stocked full of the amino acid leucine. Dr. Donald Layman has proved that leucine enhances lean muscle tissue and lower body fat levels.

Whey protein can assist in weight loss, but it's important to understand that there is nothing particularly magical about whey protein that will cause you to melt off those pounds of belly fat. In fact, the goal of drinking whey protein is usually to add or preserve muscle weight, not to lose it. With whey you can change your body fat percentage to favor lean tissue. Including whey protein along with resistance training will help you become leaner overall … and yes, that will include losing some belly fat.

When buying a whey protein product, "Whey Protein Isolate" is the highest quality you can buy; which has at least 90 percent protein with only trace amounts of fat and lactose. Also check the sugar count; some brands add way too much sugar to make whey taste like candy and get you hooked on their product…and that sugar isn't going to help our waist line! If you do decide to try whey protein powder, it's important to read the ingredients on the product closely. Some whey protein powders have added ingredients that can be counter-productive to your goals. For example, whey protein "gainer" powders have tons of extra calories added to them in the form of sugar in order to increase their calorie content for people who are trying to gain weight. Jay Robb is a superior weight loss brand that uses stevia to sweeten their whey.

There are many ways to consume whey protein. I personally like to "chew my food" so I add it to my baked goods. It can also easily be added to water, almond milk, cottage cheese, or used as an egg replacement in many baking recipes. For baking ideas such as chocolate chip cookies, animal crackers, bread sticks…check out my cookbook "Nutritious and Delicious".

Medications and Prescriptions

Are you depressed? Anxious? Can't sleep? Have allergies? On birth control? Very few people that meet are not on any prescription medications. Every medication depletes some vitamin or mineral in our body. Be aware that they can interrupt our body's delicate balance. Almost every prescription medication depletes B-vitamins from our bloodstream.

This chart is another way to discover if drugs are the root of your weight loss struggle. I'm not recommending discontinuing your prescriptions, but being aware that there are other alternatives out there. Such as when it comes to depression, it often can be an overabundance of the mineral copper in our blood, to balance that, I would recommend 50mg of zinc per day. Most anti-depressants slow metabolism except Wellbutrin, which has been found to slightly raise metabolism. So be a detective and find the best natural or prescription medication for your body and mind.

Drugs that slow Metabolism:
Diphendydramamine: to sleep (antihistamine)
Antidepressants/Anti-anxiety Medications
Diabetes Medications
Allergy Medications
Over-the-Counter Sleep Medication
Epilepsy Medications
Migraine Medication
Hormonal Treatments: inflammation, fertility and cancer

CHAPTER 9

SPECIFIC INGREDIENTS AND PANTRY LIST

Putting it all Together!

When I shop for food, I'm not particularly interested in the "Wholesome," "Heart-Healthy" and "All Natural" claims on the front of the packages. I don't give them a second glance. I'm too busy scanning the package for the most important thing: the ingredients list. If the ingredients themselves don't meet the mark of nutritional excellence, there's really no need to even study the label. Developing this kind of no-nonsense label savvy is essential for navigating today's grocery-store environments, where many of the more than 45,000 products make healthy claims on their packaging. You have to disregard the seduction on the front of boxes.

In 2003, the Food and Drug Administration became more relaxed in its label standards, which gave the green light for food manufacturers to plaster their products with all kinds of health claims. Bright yellow tubs of margarine now claim to "maintain a healthy heart" because they contain trace amounts of vitamin E. Prego marinara sauce claims, "HEART HEALTH," that stares you in the face, but the ingredients list shows large amount of sugar. Drinks fortified with added vitamin A and antioxidants claim they 'support immune function' even though they are loaded with sugar that hinders our immune system. And cereals, like Lucky Charms,

"Trans-Fat-Free"

Even if a food label claims the product is "trans-fat-free," check the ingredients list for hydrogenated or partially hydrogenated oils. CHEETOS claim "trans-fat free," but guess what...they have trans-fat! The FDA has a loophole that allows food manufactures to make their serving size small enough to stay under the 0.5 grams of trans-fat per serving and be able to claim "trans-fat-free." Here's a scary fact, according to the Harvard School of Public Health an estimated 30,000 people die in the United States each year from coronary heart disease caused by eating hydrogenated fats.

brag they are "whole grain" and can lower risk of cancer and heart disease, even though the refined flours and sugars cause inflammation in our arteries.

Food manufacturers are masters of deception. Become a food detective to get the information you need for yourself and your family. That means you have to avoid getting distracted by false claims and look to the ingredients list for the truth. This is where you'll find the basic components of the product. The ingredients are conveniently listed in order from the most prevalent to least. It is also to keep in mind that the more ingredients you see, the less likely this is to be a good product. The more highly processed a food product is, the more additives, stabilizers, artificial flavors, colors and texturizers it will require to look and taste appealing.

The larger the ingredient list, the more likely the item is to have dangerous food additives. The food additive sodium benzoate has been shown to damage mitochondrial DNA; and potassium bromated is a possible human carcinogen that's been banned in other countries. Avoiding trans fats, partially hydrogenated vegetable oil, high-fructose corn syrup, artificial colors (Blue 1, Blue 2, Green 3, Orange B, Red 3, Red 40, Yellow 5 and Yellow 6), butylated hydroxyanisole (BHA), butylated hydroxytoluene, monosodium glutamate, autolyzed yeast extract, hydrolyzed vegetable protein, yeast extract, natural flavoring, spices, soy extract, sulfites, nitrates, and sodium benzoate are things to steer clear of if you desire a healthy metabolism and body.

Beware that many products that claim "whole grains" or even have a "Whole Grains" stamp on the package usually also contain a large quantity of processed grains. Again, you'll need to read the ingredients list on the back.

Once you've scanned the list; check out the Nutrition Facts side panel. I focus on the amount of protein and dietary fiber, because it immediately tells me something about the quality of what I'm buying. But we also must be cautious of garbage food with a lot of added fiber…Fiber One cereal bars!

Another important fact on the Nutrition Facts panel is the serving. Food manufacturers have the luxury of setting their own serving sizes, and they often make them as small as they can as a way of decreasing the supposed number of calories and carbohydrates per serving. I've seen a single cookie labeled as containing three servings…what, who stops after a third?

100 calorie snack packs are filled with junk and more than likely assist you in putting on some pounds. Eating 100 calories of quality, real food will assist you in taking off weight. Calories are mostly a concern when they're empty, meaning they don't deliver good nutrition, or when we are likely to overindulge. Don't be scared off healthy foods that are high in calories, but good for you, like nut butters. Keep focus on high-quality ingredients instead.

Indeed, the healthiest foods in the grocery store are the fresh vegetables; which offer little or no nutrition information, in part because they don't have packaging to display it. They

"Heart Check" Symbol
The American Heart Association gives its "Heart Check" symbol to foods that have 3 grams or fewer of total fat, less than 1 gram of saturated fat, fewer than 20 milligrams of cholesterol, fewer than 480 milligrams of sodium and less than a half gram of trans fat per serving. **BUT, it does not evaluate other unhealthy ingredients, such as hydrogenated oils or high-fructose corn syrup and artificial additives.** This is a huge annoyance to nutrition experts because the inflammation caused by processed flours and sugars is now known to be a far bigger offender than fat or dietary cholesterol in the artery clogging and hardening associated with heart disease. There are some apparently 'heart healthy' cereals out there with a tons of sugar. Cereal in general is a terrible way to start your day!

aren't screaming all the "heart healthy," "cholesterol-lowering," "low-calorie" claims they could rightfully justify.

Another important tip I have is to shop and cook with your kids. Teach them to shop the perimeter of the store. Show them that whole foods like fruits, veggies, legumes, nuts and seeds are some of the healthiest and best foods we can eat. Help kids understand where foods come from, and how they contribute to the health of their muscles, skin, bones, eyes, brain function, energy, moods, and overall wellbeing. In order for kids to beat the obesity epidemic, we need to assist them to understand the food-health link.

This may seem overwhelming, but have faith. Sooner or later, you will have "an aha! moment" on how to choose quality bread, tortillas, condiments and snacks. In the meantime, be patient and keep trying.

Alternative Flours and Baking Alternatives

Please note: All flours are not created equal. If you have coconut flour in the house and the recipe calls for almond flour, your finished product will not turn out.

ALMOND FLOUR: In my family we treat corn, carrots, potatoes, rice…starchy foods, as if they were sweets (starch and sugar = excess weight gain). They are all starchy carbohydrates as are the products made from them (chips, cereal, rice cakes and snacks). So we never use alternative flours made from corn, rice or potatoes. 4 grams of carbohydrates from sugar or starch becomes 1 teaspoon of sugar in our body!

Baking with almond flour requires using more eggs to provide more structure. Use it in cakes, cookies, and other sweet baked goods. I buy mine at http://store.honeyvillegrain.com/

It is important to use **blanched almond flour**. Most recipes will not work with unblanched; most almond meal (found at Trader Joe's) is made with unblanched almonds. Unblanched means the dark outside is on the almond; it created a different texture in baking, which doesn't work as well to create soft baked goods. It makes a fine cookie, but it won't be as soft as a baked item made of 'white flour.' Here are some additional benefits of substituting almond flour for white flour:

1. DEPRESSION: Almonds contain tryptophan. This amino acid helps with serotonin production (the "feel good" chemical in the brain). When levels of serotonin fall, your body senses starvation. To protect itself, your body starts to crave carbohydrates. Serotonin levels fall after you go too long without eating, and that encourages your body to start filling itself (lose muscle).

2. HEART HEALTH/BLOOD PRESSURE/DIABETES (MAGNESIUM): Almonds are high in magnesium. Deficiencies can cause muscle spasms, pain, insomnia and fatigue. Magnesium assists in maintaining muscle mass, nerve function, a regular heartbeat, helps our immune system, and keeps bones strong. Diabetics benefit from magnesium as it helps regulate blood sugar levels. In addition, it normalizes blood pressure, and is known to be involved in energy metabolism and protein synthesis. There has been a lot of medical interest in using magnesium to avoid and manage disorders such as cardiovascular disease, diabetes, and hypertension. Almonds contain more magnesium than oatmeal or even spinach. It is found that as magnesium deficiencies increase food cravings.

3. B-VITAMINS: These are our anti-stress vitamins. Vitamin B contents also promote healthy growth of hair as well as nails. I use almond oil on my skin everyday.

4. BONE HEALTH: 1 ounce (about 23 almonds) 20-25 almonds has more calcium than 1/4 cup of milk! A valuable snack in preventing osteoporosis. You will also build strong bones and teeth with the phosphorus in almonds.

5. CANCER: Almonds are the best whole food source of vitamin E, in the form of alpha-tocopherol, which helps prevent cancer. Using almond flour instead of white flour helps to starve the cancer from high levels of glucose on which it feeds upon.

6. FIBER: The high fiber content helps with weight loss by keeping us full and tapers blood sugar from spiking. The fiber also helps in proper digestion as well as enhancing energy levels.

7. PROTEIN: Almonds have protein. Using almond flour helps give us the protein we need to build proper bones (yes…bones need protein), helps us to focus, builds muscle and staves off sarcopenia. Sarcopenia is a natural process of losing 1% of you muscle per year starting at age 25!

COCONUT FLOUR: Coconut flour is unlike any other consisting of 14% coconut oil and 58% dietary fiber! The remaining 28% consists of water, protein, and carbohydrate. It gives baked goods a rich, springy texture **but needs a lot more liquid than other flours,** for example you only need a ½ cup coconut flour for about 6 eggs in a muffin recipe; therefore you end up with a high protein muffin rather than a high carb starch bomb. If you haven't tried coconut flour yet, here are some more excellent reasons to start:

1. LOW CARB and WEIGHT LOSS: Coconut Flour is ideal for baking. It has fewer digestible carbohydrates than other flours, and it even has fewer than many vegetables! Ideal for keeping blood sugar levels low, which helps weight loss. The high fiber content also promotes a feeling of fullness.

2. GLUTEN FREE: Coconut Flour is gluten-free and hypoallergenic. With as much protein as wheat flour, coconut flour has none of the

specific protein in wheat called "gluten". This is an advantage for a growing percentage of the population who have a wheat allergy or sensitivity (many people have without knowing it).

3. INDIGESTION: Indigestion is caused by excessive hydrochloric acid in the stomach. The acid, which sterilizes food and aids during the digestive process, is secreted by the stomach wall. Usually, the stomach wall is protected by a thick coating of mucus. Persistent high levels of acid cause this coating to break down, and the acid can attack the stomach wall, causing indigestion. Alcohol and acidic foods can further irritate the stomach wall. Coconut Flour consists of the highest percentage of dietary fiber (58%) found in any flour, which improves digestion.

4. CANDIDA, CRAVINGS and DEPRESSION: The intestines crave good bacteria which improve absorption of vitamins, decreases cravings and increases serotonin. Good bacteria flourish when we eat high-fiber quality food. Yeast causes an imbalance, letting bad bacteria in; they love sugar and starch. Yeast and bad bacteria damages the intestinal wall and produces toxic by-products which can be absorbed into the blood and sent throughout the body. This is how food allergies and leaky-gut syndrome begins.

5. PROTEIN: It is also high in protein which helps increase the Thermic Effect of Food, which increases metabolism. Protein also increases focus and mood.

6. REDUCE GALLSTONES: Gallstones form as a result of a gathering of cholesterol and salts from bile. Bile plays an important role in the absorption of fats from the intestinal tract because it makes fats soluble. Eating high fiber and low carb foods using coconut flour as well as LOTS OF WATER can decrease the chances of gallstones recurring. Galls are released by certain dietary fats. Are you or have you been on a low fat diet???

7. IBS/CROHN'S/COLITUS: Irritable bowel syndrome (IBS) is a malfunction of the nerves in the wall of the bowel that make the bowel muscle contract. It can be connected to stress, vitamin deficiencies and low serotonin levels (depression). One treatment is to consume a high fiber diet; that in combination with coconut oil (a medium chained triglyceride) is VERY helpful for IBS.

8. HEART DISEASE/STROKE/BLOOD PRESSURE: Studies have proven that coconut fiber protects against heart attacks and strokes; it helps reduce cholesterol. Even modest increases in fiber intake can also significantly reduce blood pressure.

9. NO PHYTATES: Most fibrous foods such as seeds, wheat, and oats have phytic acid. This acid causes mineral deficiencies because it binds to minerals in the foods we consume (calcium, zinc and iron). Phytic acid pulls them out of the body resulting in mineral deficiencies. Coconut fiber does not contain phytic acid so it helps improve mineral status when you replace this for wheat flour in your baked goods.

10. HEMORRHOIDS: The high fiber content can help move things along. Just remember to consume extra water when you add in fiber or things can get worse!

11. DIABETICS: Coconut Flour consists of the highest percentage of dietary fiber found in any flour. Fiber helps moderate swings in blood sugar by slowing down the absorption of sugar into the blood stream. This helps keep blood sugar and insulin levels under control.

12. CANCER: Coconut flour is fermentable and produces high amounts of butyric acid which helps in stopping tumor formation. Studies have proven that butyric acid slows the growth of tumor cells and prompt all cells to develop properly. Coconut fiber also promotes good bacteria flourish which boosts our immune system. The high fiber content acts like a broom, sweeping the intestinal contents through the digestive tract. Parasites, toxins, and carcinogens are swept along with the fiber. This prevents toxins that irritate intestinal tissues and cause cancer from

getting lodged in the intestinal tract (decreases colon cancer). Since it is low carb, it also helps people maintain a low carb/sugar diet to stop feeding the cancer glucose which the cancer "feeds" upon.

PEANUT FLOUR: As long as you don't have a problem with candida, peanut flour is a flavorful ingredient. Peanut flour is a dry powder formed after the partial removal of oil from the nut. It is used to add flavor and protein to baked goods, snacks, as well as to sauces, marinades and dressings. While peanuts are about 25% protein, peanut flour is about 50% protein. That's because the process of removing fatty oil from roasted peanuts enriches the levels of the remaining peanut components. The resulting flour is naturally low in fat, high in protein and relatively low in carbohydrates.

It is a great thickener for soups, a flavorful and aromatic ingredient for breads and pastries, as well as a creative coating for meats, fish, and other dishes. Peanut flour is a good source of Vitamin E, Folate, Fiber, Niacin, Magnesium, and Phosphorus.

Peanut flour is not self-rising and will need a rising agent added if called for in your recipe. When baking with peanut flour, you may want to add an extra egg or other moistening agent to prevent dryness.

HAZELNUT FLOUR: Using this for baked goods gives your dough a sweet nuttiness as well as fiber and iron. After first being diagnosed with a gluten allergy, you may feel tired; this is linked to an iron deficiency. I like to make my muffins with this. Nuts are considered a carbohydrate; however hazelnuts are very low in starch.

FLAXSEED: This seed has many health benefits such as high-quality protein, fiber, B and C vitamins, iron, and zinc, anti-cancer properties, omega-3 fatty acids, and many other benefits. To use as an egg substitute grind 2 tablespoons flaxseed and add 6 tablespoons boiling water. I have a chocolate flaxseed muffin in my cookbook "Nutritious and Delicious" that is a favorite of many clients.

PSYLLIUM HUSK: It is a powerful fiber that can be used in place of white flour in many baked goods. Some benefits include:

1. Maintains healthy cholesterol levels, including a proper balance of HDL and LDL cholesterol.
2. Decrease Constipation: Unlike stimulant laxatives, Psyllium husks are gentle and are not habit forming. Psyllium husks' bulking action makes elimination easier and more comfortable.
3. Reduce Toxins and Estrogen Dominance = Psyllium sweeps waste, excess estrogen and toxins more quickly out of the body, so toxins are not reabsorbed from the colon back into the bloodstream.
4. Reduces the risk of getting colon cancer and hemorrhoids, alleviate bladder and kidney problems, help lower blood glucose in diabetics, help to make labor easier by dilating the cervix, and help dieters lose more weight.
5. Natural Antibiotic: It is sold as a cough syrup in many parts of the world. In Argentina it is brewed and strained, then chilled and used to reduce inflammation. In India it is used to treat rheumatism and gout in a mixture of oil and vinegar. Old World remedies used psyllium seeds in a poultice to treat wounds and sores.
6. Gluten-Free: Psyllium husks do not contain any gluten so people who are gluten sensitive can use them.

Flour Substitutions (Per Cup)					
FOOD	Rate	Carbs	Sugars	Fiber	Calories
Rice Flour (GLUTEN-free foods)	Bad	127	0.2	3.8	578
White Flour	Bad	100	0	4	496
Wheat Flour	bad	87	0	14	407
Oat Flour	bad	78	0	12	480
Almond Flour	Best	24	4	12	640
Peanut Flour	Best	21	4	9	196
Coconut Flour	Best	80	0	48	480
Flaxseed meal	Best	32	0	32	480
Psyllium Husks	Best	51	0	51	132

GUAR GUM/XANTHAN GUM: If you are new to baking gluten free baking you may be thinking "What is the Xanthan Gum and Guar Gum?" and "Why do I need them?" To put it simply, they help keep your mixes mixed, they keep oil droplets from sticking together or separating, and solid particles from settling to the bottom (like when the blueberries sink to the bottom of a coffee cake). Either one works great. You can use just one or the other; but for the best results, you can use a little of both. AND I say "a little" because "a little" goes a long way! It is also used as a thickener instead of cornstarch.

The gluten in white flour creates a paste when you mix it with water (in Poland, they use this to hang wallpaper!) This sticky concoction serves the same purpose that guar gum and xanthan gum do in gluten free baking. One component of gluten free flours lack is that "chewy texture" that we crave when eating breads, adding this will help bring that texture back. Gluten protein helps thicken dough and traps air bubbles to make baked goods light and fluffy. Xanthan gum tends to help starches combine to trap air, while guar gum helps keep large particles suspended in the mix.

Guar gum is good for cold foods ("healthified" pancake syrup) while xanthan gum is better for baked goods. Foods with a high acid content (such as lemon juice) can cause guar gum to lose its thickening abilities. If all you have is guar gum when you are making a citrus baked good, just increase the amount of guar gum.

HELPFUL TIP: Add thickener to the oil in a recipe, making complete mix of oil and gum before adding to the rest of liquid ingredients. Using a blender or a food processor helps get them to dissolve properly; clumps will make a big unappetizing bite in foods. *NOTE: people with severe allergies should use guar gum.

CONVERSION for Gluten Free Flour

Cookies......1/4 tsp Xanthan gum OR ½ tsp Guar Gum per cup of flour

Cakes and Pancakes.........1/2 tsp Xanthan gum OR 3/4 tsp Guar Gum per cup of flour

Muffins and Quick Breads.....3/4 tsp Xanthan Gum OR 1 tsp Guar Gum per cup of flour

For Liquids (salad dressing/soups).....1/2 tsp Xanthan Gum per 8 oz OR 1-3 tsp guar gum per 1 quart of liquid

ALMOND FLOUR VS COCONUT FLOUR PUMPKIN DONUT

1 ½ cups blanched almond flour	1/2 cup coconut flour
¼ tsp Celtic sea salt	1/4 tsp Celtic sea salt
½ tsp baking soda	1/4 tsp baking soda
3 large eggs	6 eggs
½ cup Just Like Brown Sugar	1/2 cup Just Like Brown Sugar
1 tsp cinnamon	1 tsp cinnamon
1 tsp pumpkin pie spice	1 tsp pumpkin pie spice
2 TBS Butter or Coconut Oil	2 TBS coconut oil or butter
1 cup fresh pumpkin	1 cup fresh pumpkin

In a mixing bowl combine almond/coconut flour, baking soda, salt, and spices. Mix butter, sweetener, eggs and pumpkin until smooth. Stir wet ingredients into dry (Add ½ tsp guar gum). Grease donut pan. Spoon batter into the pan. Bake at 325° for 30-40 minutes.

If you crave sweets while trying to conquer addictions to tobacco and alcohol then the sweetness of these alternative sweeteners can help to fulfill these cravings in a healthy manner and not play havoc with weight and blood sugar. Here are the natural sweeteners I use and why.

STEVIA GLYCERITE

Stevia glycerite is a favorite of many people. It is an herb that has been used as a sweetener in South America for hundreds of years. One tip is to look for "stevia glycerite;" which has no bitter aftertaste as compared to plain "stevia." It is widely used all over the world. In Japan, it claims 58% of the sweetener market, and was used in Japanese Diet Coke until the company replaced it with aspartame to "standardize" worldwide.

CALORIES
0

CONVERSION
300 times sweeter than sugar. 1 tsp of stevia = 1 cup of sugar

WHY I USE IT
It is great for cooking, because it maintains flavor that many other sweeteners lose when heated, but it also needs an additional sweetener in most cases when making baked goods since it doesn't caramelize or create "bulk."

BENEFITS OF STEVIA
1. WEIGHT LOSS and DIABETICS: It does not affect blood sugar metabolism. This makes it a great tool in weight loss programs, but it also for diabetics. Stevia creates a hypoglycemic effect and increases glucose tolerance. It significantly decreases plasma glucose levels. In multiple human studies, blood sugar is reduced by 35% 6-8 hours after consumption of a hot water extract of the leaf.

2. BLOOD PRESSURE: Stevia extract is a vasodilator agent. Studies show that a mix of hot water and extract from the leaf lowers both systolic and diastolic blood pressure. Several studies demonstrated this hypotensive action (as well as a diuretic action).

3. ANTI-BACTERIAL/ANTI-YEAST: has anti-bacterial properties in that it helps to inhibit the growth and reproduction of harmful bacteria

that lead to disease. It helps prevent dental cavities by inhibiting the bacteria Streptococcus mutans that stimulates plaque growth. It also has vaso dilatory activity and is effective for various skin issues, such as acne, heat rash, and problems caused by insufficient blood circulation.

4. CANCER: It keeps your body in a ketogenic state so you can starve the cancer of sugar on which cancer feeds upon.

UNDESIRED PROPERTIES = It doesn't create a "caramelized" cookie, or "bulk" in baked goods, which is why I add erythritol.

ERYTHRITOL (PREFERED BRAND = ORGANIC ZERO)

Erythritol is a naturally-derived sugar substitute that looks and tastes very much like sugar, yet has almost no calories. Erythritol has been used in Japan since 1990 in candies, chocolate, yogurt, fillings, jellies, jams, beverages, and as a sugar substitute. Erythritol, is considered a 'sugar alcohol' and is found naturally in small amounts in grapes, melons, mushrooms, and fermented foods such as wine, beer, cheese, and soy sauce. Erythritol is usually made from plant sugars.

CALORIES
0 to 0.2 calories/gram (95% fewer calories than sugar)

CONVERSION
70% as sweet as table sugar. Use cup for cup like sugar, but you need to add a tsp of stevia glycerite to add sweetness.

WHY I USE IT
Unlike stevia, it has a crystallization property like sugar. This is why it is combined with stevia for baking.

BENEFITS OF ERYTHRITOL
1. WEIGHT LOSS and DIABETES: Erythritol does not affect blood glucose or insulin levels.

2. ORAL HEALTH: Erythritol isn't metabolized by oral bacteria which break down sugars and starches to produce acids, which means that it doesn't contribute to tooth decay. This is why excess carbohydrates and table sugar lead to tooth enamel loss and cavities formation.

3. CANDIDA: Erythritol is absorbed in the small intestines, which reduces fermentation and decreases the detrimental problems associated with Candida (yeast overgrowth in the body).

UNDESIRED PROPERTIES = It doesn't dissolve in foods (like salad dressings/caramel)

NAME BRANDS OF STEVIA AND ERYTHRITOL COMBINATIONS

TRUVIA

Coca-Cola now has a sweetener composed of stevia and erythritol.
CONVERSION
Same as sugar.
CALORIES
0.2 calories/gram
BEFEFITS and UNDESIRED PROPERTIES
Same as erythritol and stevia (see above). It also is expensive and I don't enjoy opening a million little packets if the store doesn't carry the tubs! This is why I purchase erythritol and stevia glycerite separate and mix my own!

ZSWEET

Is another brand of a erythritol and stevia mix. It comes in convenient large bags (as compared to the small tubs of Truvia). A lot of people prefer the taste of ZSweet over other non-caloric sweeteners.
CALORIES
0
CONVERSION
Same as sugar.
BENEFITS/UNDESIRED PROPERTIES
Same as stevia and erythritol.

ORGANIC ZERO

Is produced from Organic Sugar Cane Juice, which is naturally fermented and crystallized to create Organic Erythritol.
CALORIES
0.2 cals/gram
CONVERSION
Organic Zero is 70% as sweet as table sugar. You need to add 1 tsp of stevia to your baked goods when using Organic Zero.

BENEFITS

Same as erythritol. And baked goods made with Organic Zero have longer "shelf lives" than those made with regular sugar.

UNDESIRED PROPERTIES

The molecular structure of Organic Zero prevents it from browning the way other sugars do.

XYLITOL

Xylitol occurs naturally in many fruits and vegetables and is even produced by the human body during normal metabolism. Manufacturers make it from plants such as birch and other hard wood trees and fibrous vegetation. Some people prefer the taste of xylitol. I only use it when I have to due to since it has a higher calorie content and causes an increase in insulin. Before I found JUST LIKE SUGAR, I used this for my caramel sauce.

CALORIES

2.4 calories/gram; 1 tsp has 9.6 calories and 1 tsp of sugar has 15 calories (40% fewer calories and 75% fewer carbs than table sugar)

CONVERSION

Same as table sugar. Use cup for cup.

BENEFITS

1. REDUCES CAVITIES: It does not break down like sugar and keeps a neutral pH level in the mouth. Sugar produces an acidic environment in the mouth, which increases bacteria and weakens the enamel protecting the teeth. Xylitol prevents bacteria from sticking to the teeth, which protects the teeth from tooth decay. After eating xylitol, acid-producing bacteria falls as much as 90%, therefore the bacteria can't stick to the surface of the teeth which decrease plaque buildup.
2. REDUCES EAR INFECTIONS: It has be used as medicine for ear infections because it clears out excess earwax and inhibits the growth of harmful bacteria in the pharyngotympanic tubes.
3. HELPS WITH ASTHMA: Since asthma is linked to chronic post-nasal drip, xylitol helps by breaking the cycle of bronchial inflammation.
4. CLEARS UP CANDIDA: Candida is an opportunistic fungus which feeds on sugars and other yeast-containing foods (foods that are aged, pickled, dried, fermented or cured).
5. BOOSTS IMMUNE SYSTEM: Xylitol increases our White Blood Cells, therefore boosting our immune health and protects us from chronic disease and bacterial infections.

6. STREPTOCOCCUS: Protects newborns from streptococcus if the nursing mother consumes this. It is proven to help decrease this oral bacteria by 80%.

7. DECREASE ALLERGIES AND SINUS INFECTIONS: They now have a nasal spray made of xylitol because it decreases the harmful bacteria that gather in the cells of our nose.

8. REDUCES OVARIAN CYSTS, PCOS and BREAST CANCER: Consuming sugar creates high insulin levels which increase the production of estrogens, leading to an estrogen-dominant condition, and also interfere with healthy ovarian function. Insulin resistance is a major cause of a growing hormonal problem called polycystic ovarian syndrome (PCOS). Signs that the body is being exposed to higher levels of the male hormones include acne, loss of head hair, and an increase in body hair. Lowering insulin levels is crucial for not only treating PCOS but also resolving most other hormonal imbalances, including those leading to breast cancer. Xylitol is a natural insulin stabilizer. There are no sharp rises and falls in insulin levels such as occur with sugar.

UNDESIRED PROPERTIES

Xylitol has very few known side effects, although some people report diarrhea when adding xylitol into their diets.

JUST LIKE SUGAR

It is made from chicory root, calcium, vitamin C, and orange peel.

CONVERSION

Same as table sugar. Use cup for cup.

CALORIES

0

WHY I USE IT

Just Like Sugar has none of the strong aftertaste of stevia or artificial sweeteners.

BENEFITS

Keeps ice cream soft, makes perfect caramel sauce, makes cookies soft on the inside and chewy on the outside, it tastes great...shall I go on?

1. CHOLESTEROL: It decreases the levels of serum LDL cholesterol in the blood.

2. INFLAMMATION: It contains vitamin C, one of the most powerful antioxidants.

3. DIABETES: The inulin content is not digestible, so its lack of glucose can help promote optimal blood sugar levels while also increasing stool

bulk and consistency.

4. CONSTIPATION: It provides soluble fiber, which improves digestion.

5. GALL BLADDER ISSUES: It builds your body's resistance to gallstones and liver stones. By increasing the flow of bile, it assists the body in digesting foods and liquids. The extra bile also helps break down fats in the body. Chicory root has a mild laxative effect, increases bile from the gallbladder, and decreases swelling.

6. URINARY INFECTIONS, KIDNEY STONES and GOUT: It has diuretic properties that provide protection for the urinary tract system and kidneys. Toxins are removed and the cleansing of the body is stimulated because of an increase in urine flow. It has been used to expel gravel, calcium deposits, and excess uric acid from the body, which helps to prevent gout and kidney stones.

7. WEIGHT LOSS: Chicory root benefits weight loss because of the effect it has on the digestive system. It is an excellent source of fructooligosaccharides which help promote the growth of beneficial bacteria in your digestive tract. It also increases the rate of the breakdown of fats. It also helps with weight loss because it helps keep insulin levels low while enjoying sweet foods.

8. NATURAL "Liver" CLEANSER: Chicory root also supports the body's detoxification system through the liver and kidneys, and is believed to help with calcium absorption. Chicory also helps prevent jaundice and an enlarged liver when mixed with water. Because of Chicory Root's potential for removing contaminants from the digestive system, the liver does not have to work as hard to filter out toxins that may have escaped into the bloodstream. It also acts as a gentle laxative and diuretic for removing excess water and toxins, and this can also reduce strain on the liver.

9. ANXIETY: It is a natural sedative and anti-inflammatory for the nervous system. If you have anxiety issues and still drink coffee, this sweetener can help.

10: INDIGESTION: It acts as an herbal antacid, the root neutralizes acid and correct acid indigestion, heartburn, gastritis, vomiting, upset stomach. Because it stimulates bile production, this helps to speed up the digestive process after eating too much rich food.

UNDESIRED PROPERTIES

It is expensive, but other than that it is perfect!

If you read labels you might see ingredients like oligofructose and inulin starting to show up on food packages. These 2 words are called 'prebiotics' in the nutrition world. Prebiotics are non-digestible foods that make their way through our digestive system and help good bacteria grow and flourish. Prebiotics keep beneficial bacteria healthy. They are found in small amounts in many plants. Plants with large amounts of oligosaccharides include chicory root. About 90% makes it past digestion in the small intestine and reaches the colon where it performs a different function: that of a prebiotic.

Just Like Sugar contains 96 grams of inulin fiber per cup! The ingredients of Just Like Sugar = Chicory Root, Calcium and Vitamin C.

Prebiotics help increase probiotics, which are beneficial bacteria that help keep your digestive system healthy. The majority of my clients have malfunctioning digestive systems for a variety of reasons. Our typical 'Western' eating habits and stress can all negatively impact the 'good bacteria' in our gut. Probiotics are helpful micro-organisms that live in our intestinal tract. In a healthy body, good bacteria make up most of the intestines' micro-flora and protect digestive health. If you have primarily good bacteria, your immune system will function optimally and it will help you extract essential nutrients in the foods you eat. In order to feed our cells, we need to absorb the nutrients from our food, otherwise our brain will keep telling us to eat until the cells are fed.

Here are the most common warning signs of a bacterial imbalance, if you suffer one or more of these problems it is quite likely that eating prebiotics and taking a probiotic supplement could help you get your 'system' back on the right track:
1. Allergies and food sensitivities
2. Difficulty losing weight, sugar/carbohydrate craving
3. Frequent fatigue, poor concentration
4. Frequent constipation or diarrhea

5. Faulty digestion, acid reflux and other gut disorders
6. Sleeping poorly, night sweats
7. Painful joint inflammation, stiffness
8. Bad breath, gum disease and dental problems
9. Frequent colds, flu or infections
10. Chronic yeast problems
11. Acne, eczema skin and foot fungus
12. Extreme menstrual or menopausal symptoms

There are many stresses and factors that can kill your 'friendly bacteria' every day. Here is a summary of some of the commonest good-bacteria-KILLERS:
1. Antibiotics
2. Birth control pills
3. Steroidal & hormonal drugs
4. Fluoride (added to toothpaste and sometimes to drinking water!)
5. Chlorine (added to water to kill bacteria...it kills friendly-bacteria too!)
6. Coffee/Tea
7. Carbonated drinks
8. Stress
9. Preservatives
10. Additives (colorings, flavorings and chemicals in processed foods)
11. Pesticides (choose ORGANIC fruit and veggies to avoid this!)
12. Fertilizers (choose ORGANIC fruit and veggies to avoid this!)

Our moods are directly correlated to the intestinal flora of our gut...the nervous system actually come from the gut to the brain; in the past scientists thought the nervous system ran the other way. This is why what we put in our stomach is so essential to our mental health. Having healthy intestinal flora; which you can achieve with probiotics and fermented foods, increase our moods and decrease our cravings. To read more on Probiotics and Cravings, check out my book Secrets to Controlling Your Weight Cravings and Mood.

So BRING on the JUST LIKE SUGAR! CHOCOPERFECTION Chocolate Bars are sweetened with Chicory Root.

Stevia Glycerite = 0
Erythritol = 0
Truvia/ZSWEET = 0
JUST LIKE SUGAR = 0
Xylitol = 7
Maple Syrup = 54
Honey = 62
Table Sugar = 68
High Fructose Corn Syrup = 100

STEER CLEAR OF:

ASPARTAME

If there is one sweetener to steer clear of Aspartame is the one. I love how the host of "Livin' La Vida Low Carb," Jimmy Moore, calls is "Nasty-tame." Aspartame was approved by the FDA in 1981 for uses in 'blue packet' tabletop sweeteners, diet soda, chewing gum, breakfast cereals, gelatins, and puddings. It can now be found in more than 6,000 foods. Aspartame is the product in NutraSweet, Equal, and Sugar Twin. It does provide calories, but because it is 160 to 220 times sweeter than sucrose so the caloric intake is negligible. The amount of aspartame in some common foods is:

- 12 oz. diet soda—up to 225 mg of aspartame
- 8 oz. drink from powder (Crystal Light)—100 mg of aspartame
- 8 oz. yogurt—80 mg of aspartame
- 4 oz. gelatin dessert—80 mg of aspartame
- ¾ cup of sweetened cereal—32 mg of aspartame
- 1 packet of Equal—22 mg of aspartame
- 1 tablet of Equal—19 mg of aspartame
- "Flinstone" Vitamins

Aspartame has been found to "eat" tiny holes in our cellular membrane. When this happens, things like Multiple Sclerosis (MS), cancer, mood disorders and many other serious issues will show up.

One woman in particular has written a book about her story with aspartame. She LOVED her diet Coke. She drank 6 cans a day. As an adult, she developed MS; which became so severe she was bound to a wheelchair. After doing some research on aspartame, she decided to kick her addiction to soda. Guess what? Her body started to heal. She is no longer in a wheelchair. She still has symptoms, but her diagnosis went from "extreme MS" to "moderate!"

Most people I meet say, "I don't have depression, but I do feel lousy, crabby, and "fly-off the handle" over no reason lately." My first suggestion is to kick the aspartame from our lips, which can be very difficult, but in the end, they become a happier person.

SPLENDA

Sucralose, also known as Splenda, is a newer sweetener on the market. It is most well known for its claim to be made from sugar. It is 600 times sweeter than table sugar. It provides basically no calories and is not totally absorbed. In 1999, it was given approval for use as an all-purpose sweetener. It is currently found in over 4,500 products, including foods that are cooked and baked. The FDA reviewed studies in human beings and animals and determined that sucralose does not cause reproductive or neurological risk to human beings.

The product Splenda is also not actually calorie-free. Sucralose does have calories, but because it is 600 times sweeter than sugar, very small amounts are needed to achieve the desired sweetness; but this is only when you use the true form (liquid sucralose). Splenda, however, is bulked-up so it can be used in place of sugar. The first two ingredients in Splenda are dextrose and maltodextrin, which are carbohydrates that are not free of calories. **One cup of Splenda contains 96 calories and 32 grams of carbohydrates, which is substantial especially for those with diabetes but overlooked due to the label claiming that it's a no calorie sweetener.**

Splenda has also been found to inhibit zinc and iodine from being absorbed, which are essential for proper thyroid function. It is also linked to decreasing good gut-bacteria, which will increase Irritable Bowel Syndrome.

THE BEST CHOICE

The best choice is to be your own detective. If you believe that you are experiencing any of the symptoms from the consumption of an alternative sweetener, then eliminating them from your diet is the best way to determine if it's so. We can't eat unlimited amounts, but a little in your coffee can save hundreds of calories which adds up to those unwanted pounds. Sweeteners are not essential nutrients in our diet, so they exist to nurture our sweet tooth, not our bodies.

13 Substitutions to control our Blood Sugar Levels

SPAGHETTI

Substitute: Spaghetti squash for spaghetti OR Fresh Shredded ZUCCHINI
Cooked spaghetti squash is Mother Nature's spaghetti. Squash has a flesh that has noodle-like strands. Cut the squash in half and remove the seeds. Then place each half (cut side down) on a plate with a quarter cup of water. Microwave the squash for 8 to 10 minutes or until it's soft to the touch. Let it cool, then scrape out the "spaghetti" strands and top with low sugar marinara sauce and cheese.
Carbohydrates Eliminated: Squash = 30 g per cup! Zucchini = 40 g per cup!
The Taste Test: "Great. Spaghetti squash has exactly the same consistency as real pasta."

PANCAKES

Substitute: Vanilla whey Protein OR Coconut Flour and cottage cheese
Place a quarter cup of whey or coconut flour and a quarter cup of cottage cheese (check for extra sugars!), two eggs, and a dash each of pure vanilla extract, and cinnamon in a blender. Mix in the blender until smooth. Cook the mixture like a regular pancake.
Carbs Eliminated: Over 45 g per pancake! Plus a bonus of an increase in

protein and fiber!

The Taste Test: "With Maria's homemade syrup, you could never tell the difference."

MACARONI AND CHEESE

Substitute: Hearts of Palm for macaroni

Not that I ever suggest making "instant" food (totally over-processed junk), but even instant mac and cheese can become a little healthier; use only half the macaroni in the box and replace it with a couple of cups of Hearts of Palm. You can find these in a jar. I replace all my noodles with these.

Carbohydrates Eliminated: 30 g per cup

The Taste Test: "If you par-boil the Palms, they taste a lot like noodles!"

PASTA SALAD

Substitute: Mixed vegetables for the pasta

Same idea as the macaroni and cheese, but try zucchini, eggplant, cauliflower, diced tomatoes, and chunks of ham, tuna, chicken, or hard-boiled eggs. Think of pasta salads as a blank canvas that you can create a beautiful and colorful spread with. Some ideas are to top them with a creamy blue-cheese dressing, a low-sugar dressing, or lime juice and slices of avocado.

Carbs Eliminated: 10 g per cup

The Taste Test: "Awesome. I don't miss the extra pasta at all. I think it actually added more flavor. If you think about it…pasta doesn't have any flavor!"

HASH BROWNS

Substitute: Squash or Shredded Cabbage for potatoes

Yellow summer squash tastes comparable to potatoes when cooked, but has just a tiny fraction of the starchy carbohydrates. To create this yummy dish, grate the summer squash, mix in an egg to use as a binder, make patties, and fry them in olive oil.

Carbohydrates Eliminated: About 15 grams (g) per hash-brown patty

The Taste Test: "Not as firm and crispy as regular hash browns, but the potato flavor is there."

MASH POTATOES

Substitute: Cauliflower for potatoes
Hardly anyone can tell the difference with this one. Steam some fresh or frozen cauliflower in the microwave (I suggest microwaving for steaming because it keeps more of the vitamins and minerals in the veggies). Then add a dash of butter to the cauliflower, add a little chicken broth or heavy whipping cream (depends on how many calories you want), and puree in a food processor or blender. Add sea salt and pepper to taste and you've got something that can compete with the real thing. To make it even better, try adding roasted garlic, cheese, or sour cream to the mixture. If you are apprehensive about your family liking this, just substitute ½ the potatoes for cauliflower the first time and see if anyone says anything!
Carbohydrates Eliminated: 30 g per cup
The Taste Test: "After a couple of bites, you forget it's not potatoes."

LASAGNA

Substitute: Zucchini or eggplant slices for noodles
Slice four to five medium-size zucchini lengthwise into three-quarter-inch-thick strips. Sprinkle Italian seasoning on the strips, place them in a single layer on a nonstick cookie sheet, and bake at 425 degrees F for 20 minutes. You want them firm, not crisp (this will get rid of any extra water). Then create the lasagna as you normally would, replace lasagna noodles with the baked zucchini.
Carbs Eliminated: 36 g per serving
The Taste Test: "Delicious. The zucchini provides texture that you don't get from noodles alone."

SANDWICHES

Substitute: Napa or Chinese cabbage for bread
Slap your turkey and Swiss onto a leaf of cabbage and roll it up. One option is to make a great-tasting BLT using cabbage instead of bread. Dip the roll in olive oil mayonnaise or mustard. My favorite is a Ruben wrap with no-sugar added Thousand Island dressing.
Carbs Eliminated: 29 g per sandwich
The Taste: "A fun way to add in a bunch of 'roughage'."

SCALLOPED POTATOES

Substitute: Tempeh or the stem of a cauliflower for potatoes

Some people automatically claim they don't like tofu, but that could be because they don't cook it right. Tempeh takes on whatever flavor you give it. I love it because it is a blank canvas and can be jazzed up with herbs and spices; it's a great substitute for potatoes. To make scalloped potatoes, sauté a couple of cups of thinly diced tempeh with garlic and onions. Then pour a cheese sauce (the sharper the better) over the tempeh cubes and bake for half an hour.

Carbs Eliminated: 11 g per cup

The Taste Test: "Just like a slightly nutty baked potato."

CHEESE-FLAVORED CHIPS

Substitute: String cheese for chips

Just crazy enough to work: Cut sticks of string cheese into quarter-inch-thick slices and scatter the rounds on a cookie sheet coated with Trader Joe's Olive Oil spray, leaving them an inch or two apart. Bake at 375 F for 4 to 5 minutes or until the cheese melts and turns golden brown. Let them cool, and then peel the chips off the tray.

Carbs Eliminated: Up to 90 g per serving

The Taste Test: "A great substitute and no trans-fats."

PIZZA

Substitute: Portobello mushrooms for pizza crust

Cut the gills out from the inside of the mushroom, then place the mushroom on a cookie sheet sprayed with Trader Joe's Olive Oil spray and bake for 5 to 10 minutes so it dries out slightly. Add no-sugar added marinara sauce, mozzarella, and pepperoni and whatever pizza toppings you like and broil for a few minutes until the cheese begins to melt.

Carbs Eliminated: About 20 g per slice

The Taste Test: "Awesome! Just like pizza, but without the guilt. Give me a fork!"

BEEF-A-RONI

Substitute: Eggplant for pasta

Mix in diced eggplant with ground beef instead of pasta is healthier and filled with fiber. You have to soften the eggplant first. Cut it in half, sprinkle it with a little salt, and broil it for 10 to 20 minutes. Let it cool, dice it up, and mix with hamburger, tomato sauce, and spices.

Carbs Eliminated: 26 g per cup

The Taste Test: "Exactly like Hamburger Helper, my kids didn't notice a difference."

RICE

Substitute: Cauliflower Rice instead of white rice

Process fresh cauliflower with a food processor until it is the size of rice. Microwave it in a covered dish. DO NOT ADD WATER. Cauliflower absorbs water like crazy, and the "granules" will become gummy. To keep it fluffy, just let the moisture in the cauliflower do its work. Great for Mexican dishes, Asian dishes…Kids even like it.

Carbs Eliminated: 32 g per cup

The Taste: "Awesome, I like it better than white rice!"

Common Ingredients to Beware of

1. **Ortega or any pre-made taco seasoning.** These are mostly filled with corn-syrup solids and fillers. It is easy and cheaper to make your own!

   1 tsp chili powder

   ¾ tsp paprika

   ¾ tsp cumin

   ½ tsp onion powder

   ½ tsp Celtic sea salt

   3/8 tsp garlic powder

   Pinch cayenne

   Combine and add to 1 pound browned and drained ground beef. Add a little water, if desired. This will be drier than taco meat made with a commercial mix due to the lack of thickeners. It tastes just as good as the store bought kind and is a lot cheaper to make.

2. **Pre-made soup mixes.** Again, they are usually filled with corn-syrup solids and fillers. Here is my yummy and cheaper recipe.

   ONION SOUP MIX

1 TBS toasted dried onion
1/2 tsp toasted onion powder
1/2 tsp beef bouillon granules (check for fillers)
1/4 tsp salt

Mix all of the ingredients together and use in French Onion Dip or other recipes that call for onion soup mix.

3. **Cream of Chicken**, Mushroom or any variety of cream soup. If you live in Wisconsin, like me, this will be an issue with many family staples. How did we survive before Cream of Mushroom soup? There are a lot of unhealthy ingredients in these canned soups. Be a scientist and find a way to make the dish without them; there are lots of tips on the internet that other health-nuts like me have given suggestions for substitutes…using real food…real cream, real chicken. I have recipes for Cream of Mushroom/Chicken/Asparagus soups on my blog.

4. **Ketchup and BBQ Sauce**: High fructose corn syrup is the main ingredient in both of these favorites. Never use ketchup to shortcut for tomato sauce; which is common when people make meatloaf, BBQ sauce, and other comfort foods. I love ketchup, so I make my own.

5. **Marinara Sauce**: People often think this is the best choice at an Italian restaurant, but it is often filled with extra sugar. Prego even labels their marinara as HEART SMART, but it has 10 grams of unnecessary sugar in the form of high fructose corn syrup. Trader Joe's has A FEW good options, but again, be a detective; just because it is sold at Trader Joe's doesn't mean it is a perfect food item. I like to make my own marinara, cheaper and organic.

6. **Cheese**: Cheese is naturally white. WI cheddar often adds food dyes to make it yellow. Stick with cheese that is white. And NEVER use "American" cheese. That junk is one molecule away from plastic! There is a link between children with autism having an increase in symptoms after eating food dyes. Also don't buy pre-shredded cheese. Notice the difference of when it is pre-shredded and when you shred your own…the cheese you shred sticks together…the pre-shredded has man-made stuff added to it so it stays separated. Shred your own and get that unplanned activity metabolism burning.

7. **Milk**: If a recipe calls for milk, use unsweetened almond milk; regular milk has lactose sugar and is filled with hormones. Science is now

linking the early development of young girls and fertility problems in women to the hormones added to milk. Almond milk also has a little fat to help balance out blood sugar levels and only 40 calories per cup vs. 90 calories per cup for skim milk. It also comes in chocolate! Check out my tomato gorgonzola bisque recipe on my blog mariahealth.blogspot.com.

8. **Beef**: Try to always use Grass Fed Beef which is filled with Omega 3's. Corn Fed Beef in stores are filled with Omega 6's. Venison is also filled with Omega 3's. Buffalo is your best option! Buffalo and ostrich meat is leaner than chicken and filled with Omega 3's!

9. **Chicken**: When choosing chicken, try to always buy hormone-free chicken. Science is now linking the early development of young girls and fertility problems in women to the hormones added to chicken.

10. **Fiber One Products**: Yes, we want to increase our fiber, but these granola bars are glorified candy bars. Not only do they have over 20 grams of fiber, they also have as much sugar as a Snicker's bar. This increase in fiber can also cause unpleasant gas and diarrhea.

11. **Yogurt**: Unless you are buying full-fat Greek yogurt, it is not the health food the advertisers would like us to believe. Yoplait fat-free yogurt has as much sugar as a Kit Kat candy bar!

12. **Dried Fruit**: If you often suffer from migraines, dried fruit is a main culprit. Dried fruit contains sulfites and too much sugar, no fiber and minimum nutrients.

13. **Healthy Choice and other frozen dinners**: Even though they may be light in calories, they are still filled with preservatives and tons of sugar. Some Healthy Choice meals have as much sugar as a 3 Snicker's bars!!!

14. **Table Salt**: Be choosy with your salt! Table salt is nothing but junk. I only use Celtic Sea salt, which contains important trace minerals, whereas they are mostly removed from table salt. **Salt is most effective in stabilizing irregular heartbeats** and, contrary to the misconception that it causes high blood pressure, it is actually essential for the regulation of blood pressure in conjunction with water. Salt is a natural antihistamine. Salt is essential for the prevention of muscle cramps.

Fruits: Consider fruits as an occasional treat.

Good news: the fruits lowest in sugar are some of the highest in nutritional value, including antioxidants and other phytonutrients. If eating fruit for a treat try to stay in the "Fruits Lowest in Sugar" section. Remember that fructose, the sugar found in fruit, doesn't trigger our hormones to signal a "satisfied" feeling in our brain. Always include a fat and protein with fruits.

Fruits Lowest in Sugar	Apricots
Lemon or Lime	Grapefruit
Rhubarb	Fruits Fairly High in Sugar
Raspberries	Plums
Blackberries	Oranges
Cranberries	Kiwifruit
Fruits Low to Medium in Sugar	Pears
Strawberries	Pineapple
Casaba Melon	Fruits Very High in Sugar
Papaya	Tangerines
Watermelon	Cherries
Peaches	Grapes
Nectarines	Pomegranates
Blueberries	Mangos
Cantaloupes	Figs
Honeydew Melons	Bananas
Apples	Dried Fruit (Dates, Raisins, Apricots)
Guava	

Vegetables

This list is roughly arranged from lowest to highest carbohydrate.

Lowest	Peppers (Green Bell, Jalapeno)
Sprouts (bean, alfalfa, etc.)	Summer Squash
Greens – lettuces, spinach, chard, collards, mustard greens, kale	Zucchini
	Scallions or green onions
	Bamboo Shoots & Leeks
Radicchio and endive	Brussels Sprouts
Herbs - parsley, cilantro, basil, rosemary, thyme, etc.	Snow Peas (pods)
	Tomatoes
Bok Choy	Eggplant
Celery & Radishes	Artichokes
Sea Vegetables	Onions & Fennel
Cabbage/Sauerkraut	Okra
Mushrooms	Spaghetti Squash
Jicama & Avocado	Celery Root
Cucumbers (or dill pickles)	Carrots & Turnips
Asparagus	Water Chestnuts
Green/Wax Beans	Pumpkin
Broccoli & Cauliflower	Highest

STARCHY (HIGH SUGAR) VEGETABLES

The main veggies to be avoided when reducing carbohydrates are the starchier vegetables:

Beets	Potatoes in all forms
Carrots	Winter Squashes (particularly acorn and butternut)
Corn	
Parsnips	
Peas	
Plantains	

Vegetable	Carbs (1 Cup)	Fiber (1 Cup)
Artichoke	13	7
Asparagus	5	3
Avocado	11	7
Broccoli	6	2
Cauliflower	5.3	2.5
Celery	1	0.6
Cucumber	3	1
Eggplant	5	0
Green beans	5	3
Lettuce, all varieties	0 to 2	1 to 2
Peppers, all varieties	5 to 8	2 to 4
Spinach	1	1
Summer squash	1	0
Zucchini	14	6
Tomatoes	10	2
Strawberries	11	3
Raspberries	15	8
Blackberries	14	8

Vitamins and Minerals

Use this table to identify issues you may be dealing with and which vitamin and/or mineral you may be deficient in.

VITAMINS

Vitamin	What the vitamin does	Significant food sources
B1 (thiamin)	Supports energy metabolism and nerve function	spinach, green peas, tomato juice, watermelon, sunflower seeds, lean ham, lean pork chops, soy milk
B2 (riboflavin)	Supports energy metabolism, normal vision and skin health	spinach, broccoli, mushrooms, eggs, milk, liver, oysters, clams
B3 (niacin)	Supports energy metabolism, skin health, nervous system and digestive system	spinach, potatoes, tomato juice, lean ground beef, chicken breast, tuna (canned in water), liver, shrimp
Biotin	Energy metabolism, fat synthesis, amino acid metabolism, glycogen synthesis	widespread in foods
Pantothenic Acid	Supports energy metabolism	widespread in foods
B6 (pyridoxine)	Amino acid and fatty acid metabolism, red blood cell production	watermelon, tomato juice, broccoli, spinach, acorn squash, chicken breast
Folate	Supports DNA synthesis and new cell formation	tomato juice, green beans, broccoli, spinach, asparagus, okra

Vitamin	What the vitamin does	Significant food sources
B12	Used in new cell synthesis, helps break down fatty acids and amino acids, supports nerve cell maintenance	meats, poultry, fish, shellfish, cream, eggs
C (ascorbic acid)	Collagen synthesis, amino acid metabolism, helps iron absorption, immunity, antioxidant	spinach, broccoli, red bell peppers, tomatoes
A (retinol)	Supports vision, skin, bone and tooth growth, immunity and reproduction	broccoli, tomatoes, pumpkin, beef liver
D	Promotes bone mineralization	self-synthesis via sunlight, fortified milk, egg yolk, liver, fatty fish
E	Antioxidant, regulation of oxidation reactions, supports cell membrane stabilization	polyunsaturated plant oils, sunflower seeds, tofu, avocado, shrimp, cod
K	Synthesis of blood-clotting proteins, regulates blood calcium	Brussels sprouts, leafy green vegetables, spinach, broccoli, cabbage, liver

Mineral	What the mineral does	Significant food sources
Sodium	Maintains fluid and electrolyte balance, supports muscle contraction and nerve impulse transmissions	salt, Tamari sauce, meats
Chloride	Maintains fluid and electrolyte balance, aids in digestion	salt, Tamari sauce, milk, eggs, meats
Potassium	Maintains fluid and electrolyte balance, cell integrity, muscle contractions and nerve impulse transmission	artichoke, spinach, broccoli, green beans, tomatoes, avocado, meats, cod
Calcium	Formation of bones and teeth, supports blood clotting	Almonds, yogurt, cheddar cheese, Swiss cheese, tofu, sardines, green beans, spinach, broccoli
Phosphorus	Formation of cells, bones and teeth, maintains acid-base balance	all animal foods (meats, fish, poultry, eggs, milk)
Magnesium	Supports bone mineralization, protein building, muscular contraction, nerve impulse transmission, immunity	spinach, broccoli, artichokes, green beans, sunflower seeds, tofu, nuts, seeds, halibut
Iron	Part of the protein hemoglobin (carries oxygen throughout body's cells)	artichoke, parsley, spinach, broccoli, green beans, tomato, tofu, clams, shrimp, beef liver

Mineral	What the mineral does	Significant food sources
Zinc	A part of many enzymes, involved in production of genetic material and proteins, transports vitamin A, taste perception, wound healing, sperm production and the normal development of the fetus	spinach, broccoli, green beans, oysters, shrimp, crab, turkey (dark meat), lean ham, lean ground beef, lean sirloin steak, plain yogurt, Swiss cheese, tofu, ricotta cheese
Selenium	Antioxidant. Works with vitamin E to protect body from oxidation	Seafood and meats
Iodine	Component of thyroid hormones that help regulate growth, development and metabolic rate	Celtic sea salt, seafood, kelp, cheese
Copper	Necessary for the absorption and utilization of iron, supports formation of hemoglobin and several enzymes	meats, water
Manganese	Facilitates many cell processes	widespread in foods
Chromium	Associated with insulin and is required for the release of energy from glucose	liver, brewer's yeast, cheese, nuts
Molybdenum	Facilitates many cell processes	legumes, organ meats

THINGS IN MY PANTRY

Here is a helpful pantry list to follow. I suggest anyone with depression, thyroid disorder or other autoimmune diseases to stay away from gluten and grains. The items on the list with gluten will have a *symbol in front of them.

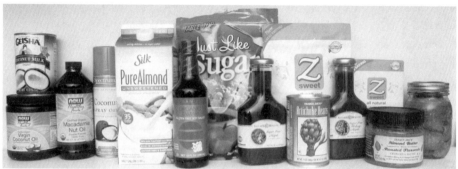

OILS
Macadamia Nut Oil
Almond Oil/Walnut Oil
Coconut Oil
Coconut Oil Spray
Sesame Oil
Pasture Fed Butter

NOODLES
Zucchini Noodles
Cabbage Noodles
Miracle Noodles

SAUCES/SPREADS/CONDIMENTS
Organic Salsa
Organic Tamari Sauce (fermented soy sauce)
Contadina Thick and Zesty Tomato Sauce
Mustard (Stone ground)
Homemade Ketchup (Option: Nature's Hollow Brand)
Homemade BBQ Sauce (Option: Nature's Hollow Brand)
Homemade Marinara Sauce (Option: Seeds of Change Marinara 4 carbs)

Hot Sauce
Pesto (made with macadamia nut oil)
Homemade Cocktail Sauce (Option: Trader Joe's)
Homemade Coconut Milk Syrup (Option: Nature's Hollow Brand)
Homemade Jelly (Option: Nature's Hollow Brand)
Spectrum Organic Mayonnaise

DAIRY
Unsweetened Almond Milk
Unsweetened Coconut Milk
Full-Fat Can Coconut Milk
REAL Whipping Cream
Sour Cream
Cream Cheese
WHITE Raw Cheddar Cheese
Cottage Cheese/Ricotta Cheese

PROTEINS
Grass-Fed Meat (hamburger/steaks)
Grass-Fed Bison and Ostridge
Free Range Eggs
Hormone Free Organic Chickens
Shrimp
Clams
Canned Crab
Homemade Canned Salmon
Smoked Salmon
Bolinski's Organic Chicken Sausage
Canned Light Tuna (Albacore has more mercury)
Canned Oysters
Canned Sardines
Applegate Farms Hotdogs
Trader Joe's Bacon (never turkey bacon!)
Homemade Jerky

SOUPS
Organic Beef Broth
Organic Chicken Broth
Organic Vegetable Broth

NUTS
Almond Butter
Almonds
Organic Natural Peanut Butter
Peanuts in the shell
Sunflower Seeds
Walnuts/Macadamia nuts
Pecans
Brazil Nuts

FRUITS and VEGETABLES
No Fruit: only organic berries and only when in season as a dessert!
Cabbage (for "pasta")
Cauliflower (for "rice")
Dark Leafy Greens
Peppers (Stuff with Sloppy Joes)
Homemade Sauerkraut
Homemade DILL Pickles
Zucchini (into "Noodles")
Kale (Kale CHIPS!)
Pumpkin (only when in season)
Artichokes (Easy Pizza Casserole)
Broccoli
Asparagus
Hearts of Palm (Tuna "Noodle" Salad)
Mushrooms (Cowboy Chicken Casserole)
Portabella Mushrooms (use as Pizza Crust)

FROZEN FOODS
Homemade Ice Cream (using Just Like Sugar)
SoDelicious No Sugar (NO-AGAVE) Coconut Milk Ice Cream
Clemmy's Ice Cream
Homemade Protein Waffles
Homemade Baked Goods

BAKING PRODUCTS and SWEETENERS
Aluminum Free Baking Powder
Baking Soda
Guar Gum/Xanthan Gum (thickener)
Stevia Glycerite
Erythritol
ZSweet
Organic Zero
JUST LIKE SUGAR
JUST LIKE BROWN SUGAR
Coconut Flour
Blanched Almond Flour
Peanut Flour
Pecan Meal/Hazelnut Meal (Pecan Sandies)
Unsweetened Cocoa Powder
Unsweetened Baking Chocolate (Maria's Chocolate Torte)
Unflavored Jay Robb Whey and Egg White Protein
Vanilla Jay Robb Whey and Egg White Protein

SPICES
Cinnamon
Celtic Sea Salt
Freshly Ground Pepper
Garlic Cloves
Tumeric (and other fresh spices)
Vanilla/Orange/Maple Extracts

DRINKS
Organic Coffee
<u>Variety of TEA BAGS:</u> Strawberry/Chocolate Hazelnut/Chai
STEAZ Bottled Tea
LaCroix Mineral Water
Zevita Soda

SWEETS/CHOCOLATE
Homemade Chocolate (Option: ChocoPerfection Bars)
Homemade Protein Bars (Option: Quest Protein Bars)
Homemade Cookies (Option: "Say Yes to Cookies")

EXTRA TIPS

ACTIVATE BROWN FAT

There are 2 types of fat in the body:

1. White Adipose Tissue (WAT): WAT is what we normally refer to as "body fat". We want to burn white fat, BUT brown fat is beneficial because it helps burn calories and burn the unhealthy WAT.

2. Brown Adipose Tissue (BAT): BAT is composed of iron-containing mitochondria (powerhouse of cells), which is best known for creating ATP (energy)...the more mitochondria = more energy!

BAT helps use excess calories for heat. If you use proper techniques, you can use BAT to your advantage so excess calories aren't stored as WAT which ends up as undesired belly fat. Cold stimulates BAT to burn excess fat and glucose for energy. This is why Michael Phelps can consume over 12,000 calories/day. He isn't just exercising a lot, the cool water of the pool stimulates BAT therefore he needs extra calories to keep from losing weight.

TIPS TO ACTIVATE BROWN FAT

1. Use ice packs on the back/neck for 30-60 minutes while relaxing at night when insulin levels are higher and more sensitive. Click HERE to find the one I like.
2. Soak your feet in cold water at night or right away in AM when you first wake up. This will stimulate heat throughout the day.
3. Suck on ice cubes throughout the day. I use mini ice cube trays and I sweeten the ice with Pina Colada Capella drops.
4. Have a snowcone for dessert with capella drops OR flavored stevia drops like Root Beer.
5. Take a cold shower upon arising.
6. Lower the temperature in your house by 5 degrees.

Drinking ice water = burn 60 calories
Sucking on 6 flavored ice cubes = burn 60 calories
Soaking feet in ice water for 5 minutes = burn 90 calories

Placing ice packs on body for 30 minutes = burn 100 calories
Lowering house temperature by 5 degrees = burn 100 calories/day
3 minute shower at 75 degrees F = burn 120 calories

Women typically have twice as much brown fat as men, so take advantage of it!!!

Intermittent Fasting

By now you understand that inflammation in the body is the true cause of disease, and that sugar and starch...even rice causes inflammation (if you didn't please start this book over☺). BUT so can over-nutrition. Numerous studies show that periodic fasting can have dramatic results not only in areas of weight loss, but in overall health as well. An article in the American Journal of Clinical Nutrition explains numerous benefits which include improvement in insulin sensitivity, decreases in blood pressure, reduction in free-radical damage to cells, protein and DNA, and weight loss. If you think about it, our ancestors didn't have access to food at 8am, 12noon, 3pm snack and 6pm dinner every day; they went through regular cycles where food was either abundant or non-existent. This contradicts the idea that your metabolism will 'slow down' causing you to gain weight if you don't eat 5 meals per day. In fact, intermittent fasting is more effective than calorie restriction at reducing insulin resistance.

WHY FAST:

1. Reduces insulin resistance: Insulin is drastically reduced in a glucagon dominant state (Imagine a "see-saw"; one goes up when the other goes down). When insulin is reduced it can't cause inflammation on tissues, which is associated with pain/fibromyalgia/heart disease/asthma/diabetes.
2. Reduces blood pressure: As your insulin level increases, so does your blood pres-sure. Insulin stores magnesium, but if your insulin receptors are blunted and your cells grow resistant to insulin, you can't store magnesium so it passes out of your body through urination. Magnesium in your cells relaxes muscles. If your magnesium level is too

low, your blood vessels will constrict rather than relax, which will raise your blood pressure and decrease your energy level.

3. Reduces triglycerides: Insulin upregulates lipoprotein lipase (or LPL, a fat-storage promoting enzyme) on fat tissue and inhibits activation on muscle cells. On the other hand, Glucagon upregulates LPL on muscle and cardiac tissue, while inhibiting activation of LPL on fat tissue.

4. Weight Loss

5. Reduces cancer: Fasting cleans out damaged mitochondria. It "turns on" certain genes that repair specific tissues that would not otherwise be repaired in times of surplus. Intermittent fasting has also been shown to reduce spontaneous cancers in animal studies, which is due to a decrease in oxidative damage or an increase in immune response.

6. Longer Life: Fasting allows certain cells to live longer (as repaired cells) during famine since it's energetically less expensive to repair a cell than to divide and create a new one.

So how do you put this into practice? There are a lot of ways.

1. The morning fast. The purpose is to not break the human growth hormone and glucagon-dominant state that is dubbed the 'fasted state.' This works best for people who do cardio in the morning or afternoon. This will keep the fat burning hormone (human growth hormone) high. Whenever you eat, insulin rises, which pushes human growth hormone down. Your body will derive energy from food sources (calories) or from body stores (glycogen, body fat, muscle). If you want to burn sugar, go ahead and eat before your workout, BUT if you want to burn fat, skip eating beforehand. It should last about 8 hours.

During the morning fast you are allowed:

-Coffee (if you don't have anxiety/adrenal fatigue/thyroid disorder)

-Tea/Water

-Small amounts of fatty acids (fish oil) but stay under 50 calories. Dietary fats have very minimal insulin secretion rates. If you are susceptible to anxiety or adrenal fatigue, I suggest a quality fish oil (click HERE to find the Krill Oil I like) to balance our brain chemistry and for its anti-inflammatory effects.

-Amino Acids, such as l-carnitine are recommended upon arising. This will help shuttle triglycerides to the mitochondria where we burn fat.

2. The Evening Fast: If you aren't exercising, I like this fast a little better because it keeps you from binging later in the day. Consume breakfast and lunch, then fast for the rest of the day until the next morning. I'm not a huge fan of Dr. Oz, but I know he often recommends skipping dinner once a week also. I recommend taking l-glutamine to help with muscles going into a catabolic state. It builds muscle: Muscle burns 50 calories/day, Fat burns only 2 (even when sleeping). There is a phenomenon called Sarcopenia, where we lose 1% of muscle/year starting at age 25. When you skimp on protein your body NEEDs amino acids to function properly so it eats your healthy muscles to get it…NOT GOOD!

3. Combination: Intermittent Fasting should last at least 8-10 hours when you are awake. One way to accomplish this is to have dinner no later than 3pm. Then for example you go to bed around 10pm (taking proper amino acids) and wake up at 6am. When you wake up, consume only calorie free liquids; such as water/green tea/coffee (decaf if adrenal/hormone issues), I take my l-carnitine at this time. I then recommend doing cardio (I like to run from 7:30-8:30am), I also recommend l-glutamine to repair muscles after a hard workout. Then eat at 9am. This would be a total of 18 hours in between meals, being awake for 10 hours in between meals.

STOP LOSING MUSCLE: If you continue to eat a high carb diet, you will continue to be a sugar burner. As you switch to be a ketone burner, aside from using fats for energy, it also prevents muscle loss because the need for glucose is reduced. Muscle tissue breakdown occurs when there is a need for glucose which exceeds the stores of glycogen. Fasting will also accomplish this. The dominant hormones in a fasted state (Human Growth Hormone, Glucagon, and Adrenaline) are responsible for catabolizing tissue and can aid in the breaking of fats from the glycerol backbone and using fat oxidation for energy instead of sugar. So by fasting and not working too hard, we derive energy in the form of fat. You can do anything for one day/week!

I have seen best results when people choose one so called "cheat day" a week. This helps with the body composition and thyroid function When we constantly eat small amounts of food, we tell our body to store more calories because you never eat enough for everyday functions of the body. An over-feeding day helps the body and hormones to be "tricked" that you eat plenty...no need to hold onto extra.

I don't call it a "cheat day" because I would like you to be choosy and pick a "healthified" dessert using alternative flours and sweeteners. If I called it a "cheat day" it sounds like anything is a go and it isn't.

My suggestion is to plan a meal, once a week (most people choose Saturday or Sunday) to over feed your body. I like to have a large meal on Sunday night finished off with a large piece of my "healthified" cheesecake.

With this said, we still want to keep insulin in check! Some tips to lower the insulin response when over eating:

1. Don't make breakfast a binge meal
   a. Eat a small protein breakfast (300 calories)
2. Consume 1 tsp of lemon juice with meals.
3. Supplements to lower Insulin
   a. Decaf green tea extract (200mg) at each meal
   b. Chromium (200mcg) at each meal
   c. 1 tsp cinnamon at each meal (or 1 capsule)
   d. Magnesium (200mg at each meal)
   e. Vitamin C (1000mg at each meal)
4. MOVE AFTER the MEAL
   a. Walk/Bike/Clean
5. Chew slowly and enjoy every bite
6. The slower it enters your body, the lower the insulin response

PROTEIN DAY

Some people have very damaged metabolisms where even low-starch veggies can cause an inability to lose weight. With these clients, we need to even cut out low-starch vegetables for 1 week. This will help eliminated water retention. When the body is retaining water, fat loss is very difficult. Choosing one day a week to eat only protein can help with weight loss because:

1. Increases Thermic Effect of Food (only "net" 70% of calories when you eat protein due to its metabolic effects)
2. Decreases water retention: When you retain water, fat loss is impossible.
3. It keeps you fuller longer
4. It builds muscle: Muscle burns 50 calories/day, Fat burns only 2 (even when sleeping)
   a. Sarcopenia: Loss 1% of muscle/year starting at age 25
   b. When you skimp on protein your body NEEDs amino acids to function properly so it eats your healthy muscles to get it….NOT GOOD!

*NOTE: If you get too hungry, drink FULL glass of water with 2 grams of l-glutamine to deter cravings and keep muscles from atrophying. Eat 30 minutes later or when hungry again.

Plan of Attack

Choose one day a week to have a Protein Only day, one day to Intermittent Fast and one day to "Over-Feed." For example:

1. Monday = Intermittent Fast (skip dinner)
2. Thursday = Protein only day (no veggies, only protein)
3. Saturday = Over-Feeding Day
4. Daily = Activate Brown Fat in some way.

GOOD LUCK

So with all of this information, I wish you luck in your journey to a healthy weight. I know this may all seem overwhelming and new, but try one new thing a week; maybe this week you will change your breakfast from cereal to eggs, next week start walking after dinner. 'Baby steps' are what worked for me. Instead of feeling overwhelmed, feel empowered by having the tools you need for a successful journey. No more deprivation diets of fat-free, man-made foods…real food, real satisfaction and a healthy metabolism.

SELECTED REFERENCES

Altena, T. S., et al. Effects of continuous and intermittent exercise on postprandial lipemia. Medicine & Science in Sports and Exercise (5cSuppl), 2003.

Almuzaini, K. S., et al. Effects of split exercise sessions on excess postexercise oxygen consumption and resting metabolic rate.can J Appl Physiol. 1998 Oct;23(5):433-43.

Barnes, Broda, and L Galton, Hyprthyroidism, The Unsuspected Illness, 1976, T Y Crowell, New York, NY

Belobrajdic DP, McIntosh GH, Owens JA. A high-whey-protein diet reduces body weight gain and alters insulin sensitivity relative to red meat in wistar rats. J Nutr. 2004 Jun;134(6):1454

Bouthegourd JC, Roseau SM, Makarios-Lahham L, et al. A preexercise alpha-lactalbumin-enriched whey protein meal preserves lipid oxidation and decreases adiposity in rats. Am J Physiol Endocrinol Metab. 2002 Sep;283(3):E565-72.

Brooks, B.M., et al. Association of Calcium Intake, Dairy Product Consumption with Overweight Status in Young Adults (1995-1996): The Bogalusa Heart Study. Journal of the American College of Nutrition, Vol. 25, No. 6, 523-532 (2006).

Cangiano, C., et al. Eating behavior and adherence to dietary prescriptions in obese adult subjects treated with 5-hydroxytryptophan. American Journal of Clinical Nutrition. 1992 Nov;56(5):863-7.

Cappon JP, et al. Acute effects of high fat and high glucose meals on the growth hormone response to exercise. J Clin Endocrinol Metab. 1993 Jun;76(6):1418-22.

Clippinger, B., et al. Comparison of Meal Frequency and Macronutrient Composition on Changes in Total and Regional Body. Medicine & Science in Sports & Exercise 38(5 S): S69-S70, 2006.

Collier, S. R,, et al. Growth hormone responses to varying doses of oral arginine. Growth Hormone and IGF Research 15(2):136-139, 2005.

Dhiman, TR. "Conjugated Linoleic Acid Content of Milk from Cows Fed Different Diets" 1999 J Dairy Sci 82:2146-2156.

Doi SQ, Rasaiah S, Tack I, et al. Low-protein diet suppresses serum insulin-like growth factor-1 and decelerates the progression of growth hormone-induced glomerulosclerosis. Am J Nephrol. Jul-Aug 2001;21(4):331-339.

Dillon EL, Sheffield-Moore M, Paddon-Jones D, et al. Amino Acid Supplementation Increases Lean Body Mass, Basal Muscle Protein Synthesis, and IGF-1 Expression in Older Women. J Clin Endocrinol Metab. Feb 10 2009.

Enig, Mary G, PhD, Trans Fatty Acids in the Food Supply: A Comprehensive Report Covering 60 Years of Research, 2nd Edition, Enig Associates, Inc, Silver Spring, MD, 1995, 148-154; Enig, Mary G, PhD, et al, J Am Coll Nutr, 1990, 9:471-86

Evans JL, Goldfine ID. Alpha-lipoic acid: a multifunctional antioxidant that improves insulin sensitivity in patients with type 2 diabetes. Diabetes Technol Ther. Autumn 2000;2(3):401-413.

Farreira M., Kreider R., Wilson M., Effects of CLA supplementation during resistance training on body composition and strength. J. Strength Conditioning Res. 1998; 33:521-7

Gaullier, J., et al. Conjugated linoleic acid induces regional-specific decreases in fat mass in a 6 months clinical trial. Experimental Biology Conference, San Francisco, 2006.

Gorelick-Feldman J, et al. "Phytoecdysteroids increase protein synthesis in skeletal muscle cells." J Agric Food Chem. 2008 May 28;56(10):3532-7.

Hall, W. L., et al. Casein and whey exert different effects on plasma amino acid profiles, gastrointestinal hormone secretion and appetite. British Journal of Nutrition 89(2):239-248, 2003.

Hall WL, Millward DJ, Long SJ, Morgan LM. Casein and whey exert different effects on plasma amino acid profiles, gastrointestinal hormone secretion and appetite. Br Nutr. 2003 Feb;89(2):239-48.

Hayes, A. and Cribb, P. J. Effect of whey protein isolate on strength, body composition and muscle hypertrophy during resistance training. Curr Opin Clin Nutr Metab Care. 2008 Jan;11(1):40-4.

Henrietta Blankson et al. Conjugated linoleic acid reduces body fat mass in overweight and obese humans. J. Nutr. 2000; 130:2943-2948

Herron, K.L., et al. "High intake of cholesterol results in less atherogenic low-density lipoprotein particles in men and women independent of response classification." Metabolism. 2004 Jun;53(6):823-30.

Hill, A.M., et al., "Combining fish-oil supplements with regular aerobic exercise improves body composition and cardiovascular disease risk factors." Am J Clin Nutr. 2007 May;85(5):1267-74.

Hill, A. M., et al. Combining fish-oil supplements with regular aerobic exercise improves body composition and cardiovascular disease risk factors. Am J Clin Nutr. 2007 May;85(5):1267-74.

Hubert H, et al, Circulation, 1983, 67:968; Smith, R and E R Pinckney, Diet, Blood Cholesterol and Coronary Heart Disease: A Critical Review of the Literature, Vol 2, 1991, Vector Enterprises, Sherman Oaks, CA

Hull JS. Sweet Poison, New Horizon Press, 2001

Isidori, A., et al.1981 A study of growth hormone release in man after oral administration of amino acids. Curr Med Res Opin 7:475-481.

Ivy, John, and Robert Portman (2004). Nutrient Timing: The Future of Sports Nutrition USA: Basic Health Publications.

Jim Stoppani "Insulin insight: the all-important hormone insulin can be your best friend or your worst nightmare. Follow these to make insulin work for you". Muscle & Fitness. FindArticles.com. 11 Sep, 2009.

Judelson, D. A., et al. Effect of hydration state on strength, power, and resistance exercise performance. Med Sci Sports Exerc. 2007 Oct;39(10):1817-24.

Kraemer, W.J., et al. The effects of L-carnitine L-tartrate supplementation on hormonal responses to resistance exercise and recovery. J Strength Cond Res. 2003 Aug;17(3):455-62

King, J. W. A comparison of the effects of interval training vs. continuous training on weight loss and body composition in obese pre-menopausal woman (thesis) East Tennessee State University, 2001.

Lambert, C.P., et al. "Effects of carbohydrate feeding on multiple-bout resistance exercise." J. Appl. Sport Sci. Res. 1991, 5:192-197.

Lang, C.H., Frost, R.A., Kumar, V., Wu, D., Vary, T.C. (2000). Inhibition of muscle protein synthesis by alcohol is associated with modulation of eIF2B and eIF4E, 3, 322-31

Layman, D.K., et al. "Egg Protein as a Source of Power, Strength, and Energy." Nutrition Today 44(1) 2009, 43-48.

Lavin JH. Int Journal Obesity Related Metabolism Disorders. Jan 1997.vol 21(1):pp 31-42.

Lemon, P., et al. "Beyond the Zone: Protein Needs of Active Individuals." Journal of the American College of Nutrition, Vol. 19, No. 5, 513S-521S (2000).

Levenhagen D. K., et al. (2001). Postexercise nutrient intake timing in humans is critical to recovery of leg glucose and protein homeostasis. American Journal Physiology, 280:E982 - E993.

MacDougall, J.D. et al. (1995). "The Time Course for Elevated Muscle Protein Synthesis Following Heavy Resistance Exercise." Canadian Journal of Applied Physiology. 20: 480-486. 269:E309-315.

Maki, K. C., et al. Green tea catechin consumption enhances exercise-induced abdominal fat loss in overweight and obese adults.J Nutr. 2009 Feb;139(2):264-70.

Maone TR. Dev Psychobiol, Mar 1990;vol 23(2):pp 179-191.

Markus CR, Olivier B, Panhuysen GE, et al. The bovine protein alpha-lactalbumin increases the plasma ratio of tryptophan to the other large neutral amino acids, and in vulnerable subjects raises brain serotonin activity, reduces cortisol concentration, and improves mood under stress. Am J Clin Nutr. 2000 Jun;71(6):1536-44.

Meeking DR, Wallace JD, Cuneo RC, Forsling M, Russell-Jones DL. Exercise-induced GH secretion is enhanced by the oral ingestion of melatonin in healthy adult male subjects. Eur J Endocrinol. Jul 1999;141(1):22-26.

Mercola J. Sweet Deception, Thomas Nelson, Inc, 2006.

Mori, T., et al. "Dietary fish oil upregulates intestinal lipid metabolism and reduces body weight gain in C57BL/6J mice." J Nutr. 2007 Dec;137(12):2629-34.

Muller D M, et al. Effects of oral L-carnitine supplementation on in vivo long-chain fatty acid oxidation in healthy adults. Metabolism. 51:1389-1391, 2002.

Norton, Layne E. and Layman, Donald K. (2006) "Leucine Regulates Translation Initiation of Protein Synthesis in Skeletal Muscle after Exercise" American Society for Nutrition Journal of Nutrition 136:533S-537S (February).

Patel, S. R., et al. Association between Reduced Sleep and Weight Gain in Women. American Journal of Epidemiology 2006 164(10):947-954.

Pinkoski, C., et al. The effects of conjugated linoleic acid supplementation during resistance training. Medicine & Science in Sports & Exercise 38(2):339-348, 2006.

PN Prinz, et al. "Effect of alcohol on sleep and nighttime plasma growth hormone and cortisol concentrations." Journal of Clinical Endocrinology & Metabolism, Vol 51, 759-764, 1980.

Powers ME, Yarrow JF, McCoy SC, Borst SE. Growth hormone isoform responses to GABA ingestion at rest and after exercise. Med Sci Sports Exerc. Jan 2008;40(1):104-110.

Rasmussen D.D., Sarkar D.K., Roberts J.L., Gore A.C. (2006). Chronic daily ethanol and withdrawl 6. Effects on rat sympathoadrenal activity during abstinence. Alcohol, 38(3): 173-177

Riechman, S. E., et al. Dietary Cholesterol and Skeletal Muscle Hypertrophy with Resistance Training: A Randomized Placebo-Controlled Trial. FASEB, 2008.

Riechman, S.E., et al. "Statins and dietary and serum cholesterol are associated with increased lean mass following resistance training." J Gerontol A Biol Sci Med Sci. 2007 Oct; 62(10):1164-71.

Spiegel, K., et al. Brief communication: Sleep curtailment in healthy young men is associated with decreased leptin levels, elevated ghrelin levels, and increased hunger and appetite. Ann Intern Med. 2004 Dec 7;141(11):846-50.

Swithers, S.E., et al. "A Role for Sweet Taste: Calorie Predictive Relations in Energy Regulation by Rats." Behavioral Neuroscience 2008, Vol. 122, No. 1, 161-173

Taheri S, Lin L, Austin D, Young T, Mignot E (2004) Short Sleep Duration Is Associated with Reduced Leptin, Elevated Ghrelin, and Increased Body Mass Index. PLoS Med 1(3): e62.

Tarpenning, KM, et al. Influence of weight training exercise and modification of hormonal response on skeletal muscle growth. J Sci Med Sport. 2001 Dec; 4(4):421-46.

The American College of Sports Medicine, the American Dietetic Association, and the Dietitians of Canada. "Nutrition and Athletic Performance," Medicine & Science in Sports & Medicine, 2000:Vol. 32, No. 12, pp. 2130 -2145.

Valimaki, M.J., Harkonen, M., Eriksson, C.J., Ylikahri, R.H. (1984). Sex hormones and adrenocortical steroids in men acutely intoxicated with ethanol. Alcohol, 1, 89-93

Vander Wal, J. S., et al. Short-term effect of eggs on satiety in overweight and obese subjects. J Am Coll Nutr. 2005 Dec;24(6):510-5

Volek, J.S., et al. "Body composition and hormonal responses to a carbohydrate-restricted diet." Metabolism. 2002 Jul;51(7):864-70.

Yoshioka, M., et al. Effects of red pepper on appetite and energy intake.Br J Nutr. 1999 Aug;82(2):115-23.

Wutzke, K. D, and Lorenz, H. The effect of l-carnitine on fat oxidation, protein turnover, and body composition in slightly overweight subjects. Metabolism 53(8):1002-1006, 2004.

INDEX

OTHER INFORMATION

Contact Maria Emmerich at:
www.marianutrition.com
MariaHealth.Blogspot.com
Facebook: Maria Mind Body Health

Maria's Cookbook: NUTRICIOUS and DELICIOUS

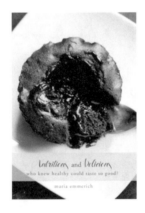

Maria's Color Cookbook Series: The Art of Eating Healthy

"Sweets" and "Kids" (more coming soon):

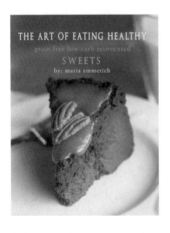
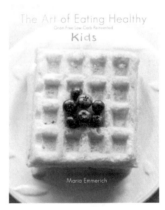